Gerda Meijler

Neonatal Cranial Ultr

M000195223

Gerda Meijler

Neonatal Cranial Ultrasonography

Second Edition

With 87 Figures and 6 Tables

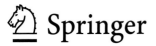 Springer

Gerda Meijler
Department of Paediatrics
Division of Neonatology
University of Toronto
The Hospital for Sick Children
555 University Avenue
Toronto Ontario, M5G 1X8
Canada
gerda.meijler@sickkids.ca

Leiden University Medical Center
Department of Paediatrics
Division of Neonatology
PO Box 9600, 2300 RC Leiden
The Netherlands
g.van_wezel-meijler@lumc.nl

ISBN 978-3-642-21319-9   e-ISBN 978-3-642-21320-5
DOI 10.1007/978-3-642-21320-5
Springer Heidelberg Dordrecht London New York

Library of Congress Control Number: 2011940857

Springer is part of Springer Science+Business Media (www.springer.com)

In memory of my father: Frits Louis Meijler, who was and still is the most inspiring person I know.

Contents

Acknowledgements

The author wants to thank:

- All the babies whose photographs and/or ultrasound scans are in this book
- The parents who gave permission to have pictures of their babies taken for educational purposes and publication
- Lise Plamondon, who, with endless patience, made the illustrations for this book and was always willing to provide repetitive adjustments
- The "Leiden group of Neonatal Neuro-Imaging": Sylke Steggerda, Sica Wiggers-de Bruïne, Annette van den Berg-Huysmans, Lara Leijser and Jeroen van der Grond for their stimulating collaboration and help
- Neonatologists and fellow-neonatologists at the LUMC for their contributions to neonatal cUS in Leiden. Neonatology, Leiden University Medical Center
- Linda de Vries and Frances Cowan for their encouragement and support

PART I

THE CRANIAL ULTRASOUND PROCEDURE

1 Cranial Ultrasonography: Advantages and Aims

1.1 Advantages of Cranial Ultrasonography

Major advantages are:

- Cranial ultrasonography (cUS) can be performed bedside with little disturbance to the infant (Fig. 1.1).
- cUS can be initiated at a very early stage, even immediately after birth.
- cUS is safe (safety guidelines are provided by the British Medical Ultrasound Society www.bmus.org and the American Institute of Ultrasound in Medicine www.aium.org).
- cUS can be repeated as often as necessary, and thereby enables visualisation of ongoing brain maturation and the evolution of brain lesions. In addition, it can be used to assess the timing of brain injury.
- cUS is a reliable tool for detection of most haemorrhagic brain lesions.
- cUS is a helpful tool for the detection of ischaemic brain lesions as well as calcifications, cerebral infections and major structural brain anomalies, both in preterm and full-term neonates.
- Some abnormalities (including lenticulostriate vasculopathy, calcifications and germinolytic cysts) are only or better detected by cUS as compared to other neuroimaging modalities.
- Doppler flow measurements of the cerebral vessels can be performed during the same examination.
- cUS is relatively inexpensive compared with other neuroimaging techniques.

G. Meijler, *Neonatal Cranial Ultrasonography*,
DOI 10.1007/978-3-642-21320-5_1,
© Springer-Verlag Berlin Heidelberg 2012

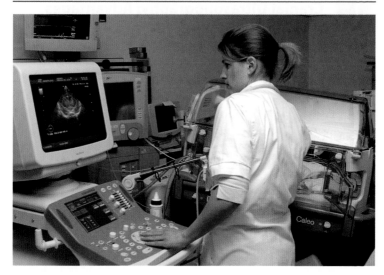

Fig. 1.1 Cranial ultrasound procedure performed in a premature infant in its incubator

- For all these reasons, cUS is an excellent tool for serial brain imaging during the neonatal period and thereafter until closure of the fontanels.

1.2   Aims of Neonatal Cranial Ultrasonography

The aims of neonatal cUS are to assess

- Brain growth and maturation
- The presence of structural brain abnormalities and/or brain injury
- The timing of injury
- The neurological prognosis of the infant

In sick neonates and in neonates with serious brain abnormalities, either congenital or acquired, cUS plays a role in decisions on continuation or withdrawal of intensive treatment. In neonates with brain injury, it may help to optimize treatment and support of the infant and its family, both during the neonatal period and thereafter.

Advantages of cUS	Aims of cUS
Safe	Exclude/demonstrate brain pathology
Bedside-compatible	Assess timing of injury
Reliable	Assess neurological prognosis
Enables early imaging	Help make decisions of intensive care treatment
Enables serial imaging	Optimize treatment and support
– brain maturation	
– evolution of lesions	
Inexpensive	
Suitable for screening	

References

American Institute of Ultrasound in Medicine. Standards for performance of the ultrasound examination of the infant brain. www.aium.org

British Medical Ultrasound Society. About Ultrasound. www.bmus.org

Further Reading

Bracci R et al (2006) The timing of neonatal brain damage. Biol Neonate 90:145–155

De Vries LS et al (2006) The role of cranial ultrasound and magnetic resonance imaging in the diagnosis of infections of the central nervous system. Early Hum Dev 82:819–825

De Vries LS et al (2004) Ultrasound abnormalities preceding cerebral palsy in high-risk preterm infants. J Pediatr 144:815–820

Govaert P, De Vries LS (2010) An atlas of neonatal brain sonography, 1st edn. MacKeith Press, Cambridge

Leijser LM et al (2006) Using cerebral ultrasound effectively in the newborn infant. Early Hum Dev 82:827–835

Lorenz JM, Paneth N (2000) Treatment decisions for the extremely premature infant. J Pediatr 137:593–595

Steggerda SJ et al (2009) Neonatal cranial ultrasonography: how to optimize its performance. Early Hum Dev 85:93–99

Van Wezel-Meijler G et al (2010) Cranial ultrasonography in neonates: role and limitations. Semin Perinatol 34:28–38

Vollmer B et al (2003) Predictors of long-term outcome in very preterm infants: gestational age versus neonatal cranial ultrasound. Pediatrics 112:1108–1114

Volpe JJ (2008a) Bacterial and fungal intracranial infections. In: Volpe JJ Neurology of the newborn, 5th edn. Saunders Elsevier, Philadelphia

Volpe JJ (2008b) Viral, protozoan, and related intracranial infections. In: Volpe JJ Neurology of the newborn, 5th edn. Saunders Elsevier, Philadelphia

Volpe JJ (2008c) Hypoxic-ischemic encephalopathy: clinical aspects. In: Volpe JJ Neurology of the newborn, 5th edn. Saunders Elsevier, Philadelphia

Volpe JJ (2008d) Intracranial hemorrhage: germinal matrix-intraventricular hemorrhage of the premature infant. In: Volpe JJ Neurology of the newborn, 5th edn. Saunders Elsevier, Philadelphia

Volpe JJ (2008e) Intracranial hemorrhage: subdural, primary subarachnoid, intracerebellar, intraventricular (term infant), and miscellaneous. In: Volpe JJ Neurology of the newborn, 5th edn. Saunders Elsevier, Philadelphia

For good-quality and safe cUS, the following conditions need to be fulfilled: a high-quality modern ultrasound machine with appropriate transducers to enable optimal image quality, and an experienced sonographer who is aware of the special needs of the sick and/or preterm neonate.

2.1   Equipment

2.1.1   Ultrasound Machine

The ultrasound machine should be a transportable real-time scanner, allowing bedside examinations without the need to transport the baby (see Fig. 1.1). It should be equipped with appropriate transducers, special software for cUS and colour Doppler flow measurements, and a storage system that enables reliable digital storage of images. Facilities for direct printing of images may be useful. Settings need to be optimised for neonatal brain imaging. It is recommended that special cUS presets be used. In individual cases and under certain circumstances, the settings can be adjusted.

2.1.2   Transducers

The use of sector or curved linear array transducers is recommended. The transducers should be appropriately sized for an almost perfect fit on the anterior fontanel (Fig. 2.1). To allow good contact between the transducer

G. Meijler, *Neonatal Cranial Ultrasonography*,
DOI 10.1007/978-3-642-21320-5_2,
© Springer-Verlag Berlin Heidelberg 2012

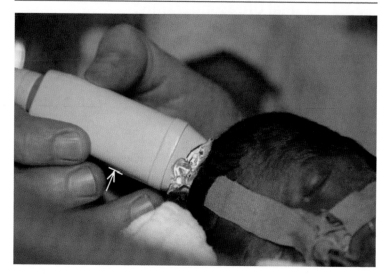

Fig. 2.1 Well-fitting ultrasound probe, positioned on the anterior fontanel. *Arrow* indicates the marker on the probe

and the skin, transducer gel is used. If the size of the fontanel allows this, we preferably use a convex (CV) transducer, as the image quality is superb compared to that of the smaller phased array (PA) probe (Fig. 2.2). If the fontanel is too small, or when hats are used for fixation of ventilatory support systems, the smaller PA probe (Fig. 2.3, see Fig. 2.1) is used. High-frequency transducers provide high near-field resolution (the higher the frequency, the better the resolution), but do not allow the same penetration as lower-frequency transducers. The ultrasound system should therefore be equipped with a multifrequency transducer (5–10 MHz) or several transducers scanning with different frequencies (5, 7.5 and 10 MHz).

In most neonates, the distance between the transducer and the brain is small, allowing the use of high-frequency transducers. High-quality images can usually be obtained with a transducer frequency set at around 7.5 MHz. This enables optimal visualisation of the peri- and intraventricular areas of the neonatal brain. For the evaluation of more superficial structures (cortex, subcortical white matter, subarachnoid and subdural spaces, superior

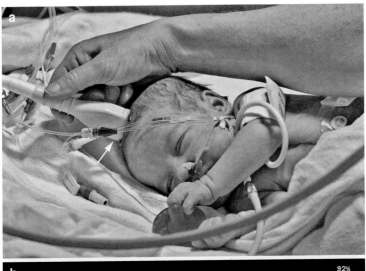

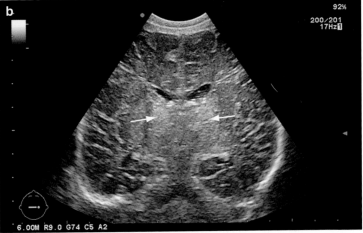

Fig. 2.2 (a) Coronal cUS scan in full-term newborn infant, scanned with the (larger) CV probe. *Arrow* indicates the marker on the probe. (b) Coronal ultrasound scan at the level of the thalami and bodies of the lateral ventricles, using the CV probe, showing increased echogenicity of the thalami (*arrows*) (full-term neonate with hypoxic-ischemic encephalopathy and deep grey matter injury)

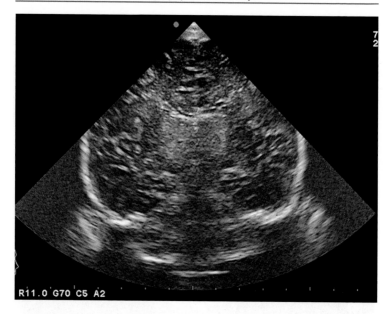

Fig. 2.3 Coronal ultrasound scan at the level of the thalami and bodies of the lateral ventricles, using the PA probe (same baby as in Fig. 2.2b)

sagittal sinus) and/or in very tiny infants with small heads, it is advised to perform additional scanning, using a higher frequency up to 10 MHz (Fig. 2.4). If deeper penetration of the beam is required, as in larger, older infants or infants with thick, curly hair or to obtain a good view of the deeper structures (posterior fossa, basal ganglia in full-term infants), additional scanning with a lower frequency (5 MHz) is recommended (Fig. 2.5). (Steggerda et al. 2009).

2.2   Data Management

Images need to be reproducible. Therefore, it is recommended that a dedicated digital storage system be used, allowing reliable storage and post-imaging assessment and measurements.

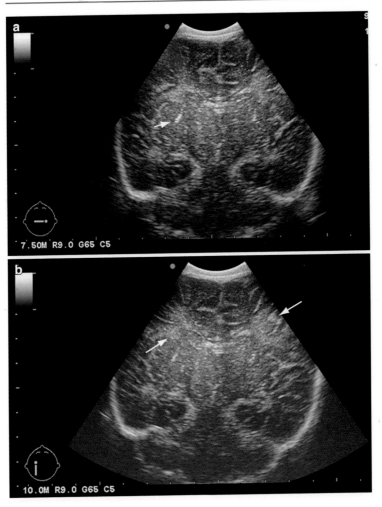

Fig. 2.4 Coronal ultrasound scans at the level of the thalami and the bodies of the lateral ventricles in full-term baby with Enterovirus encephalitis. (**a**) Transducer frequency set at 7.5 MHz. (**b**) Transducer frequency set at 10 MHZ. In (**b**), the subtle increase of echogenicity of the subcortical white matter is better depicted (*arrows*), while the basal ganglia, showing lenticulostriate vasculopathy (*short arrows*), are better depicted in (**a**)

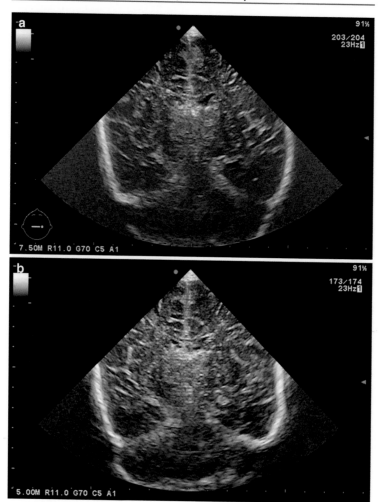

Fig. 2.5 Coronal ultrasound scans at the level of the basal ganglia and the frontal horns of the lateral ventricles in a 2½-month old baby. (**a**) Transducer frequency set at 7.5 MHz. (**b**) Decreasing the transducer frequency to 5 MHz gives better penetration into the deeper structures, but the resolution of the image is less

2.3   Sonographer and Safety Precautions

The sonographer should be specially trained to perform safe, reliable neonatal cUS examinations. In addition, he or she should be well informed with regard to the normal ultrasound anatomy and specific features of the neonatal brain and to the maturational phenomena occurring in the (preterm) neonate's brain. He or she also needs to be well informed about frequently occurring, often (gestational) age-specific brain anomalies (whether congenital or acquired) and be able to recognise these and search for them. The sonographer should be aware of the special needs of vulnerable, sick (preterm) neonates and should take the necessary hygiene precautions (including appropriate hand hygiene and cleaning of the ultrasound machine and transducers according to hospital regulations). The transducer gel should be sterile and stored at room temperature. Cooling of the infant due to opening of the incubator needs to be avoided.

cUS equipment and procedure	Transducers
• Modern, portable ultrasound machine	• 5–7.5–10 MHz
• Special cUS software	• Preferably CV probe
• Standard cUS settings; adjust when needed	• Appropriately sized
• Digital storage system	• Standard examination: 7.5–8 MHz
• Avoid manipulation and cooling of infant	• Tiny infant and/or superficial structures: use additional higher frequency (10 MHz)
• Take necessary (hygiene) precautions	• Large infant, thick hair, and/or deep structures: use additional lower frequency (5 MHz)

Reference

Steggerda SJ et al (2009) Neonatal cranial ultrasonography: how to optimize its performance. Early Hum Dev 85:93–99

Further Reading

Van Wezel-Meijler G et al (2010) Cranial ultrasonography in neonates: role and limitations. Semin Perinatol 34:28–38

3 Performing Cranial Ultrasound Examinations

Preterm neonates and sick full-term neonates are examined in their incubator while maintaining monitoring of vital functions (see also Chap. 2 and Fig. 1.1). It is recommended that the cUS examination be performed while only the incubator windows are open. Manipulation of the infant (with the exception of minor adjustments) is rarely necessary while scanning through the anterior fontanel. Older infants and full-term neonates can be examined in their cot or car seat or on an adult's lap (Fig. 3.1).

3.1 Standard Views

For a standard cUS procedure, allowing optimal visualisation of the supratentorial structures, the anterior fontanel is used as the acoustic window. Images are recorded in at least six standard coronal and five standard sagittal planes. These standard planes and the anatomical structures visualised in these planes are presented in Part II.

In addition to the standard planes, the whole brain is scanned to obtain an overview of the brain's appearance. This allows assessment of the anatomical structures and detection of subtle changes and small and/or superficially located lesions. Besides the standard views, images should be recorded in two planes of any suspected abnormality (Fig. 3.2).

3.1.1 Coronal Planes

The anterior fontanel is palpated, and the transducer is positioned in the middle, with the marker on the probe turned to the right side of the baby

G. Meijler, *Neonatal Cranial Ultrasonography*,
DOI 10.1007/978-3-642-21320-5_3,
© Springer-Verlag Berlin Heidelberg 2012

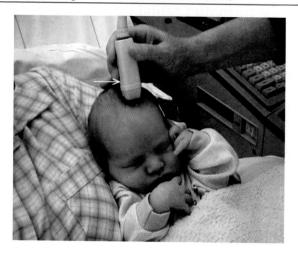

Fig. 3.1 Ultrasound examination performed in a full-term newborn infant while infant is seated on his mother's lap (*arrow* indicates marker on probe)

(see Figs. 2.1, 2.2a and 3.1). The left side of the brain will thus be projected on the right side of the monitor, and vice versa (Fig. 3.3). The probe is subsequently angled sufficiently far forwards and backwards to scan the entire brain from the frontal lobes at the level of the orbits to the occipital lobes (see Part II).

3.1.2   Sagittal Planes

The transducer is again positioned in the middle of the anterior fontanel, the marker is now pointing towards the baby's mid-face (Fig. 3.4). The anterior part of the brain will thus be projected on the left side of the monitor (Fig. 3.5). First, a good view of the midline is obtained. The transducer is subsequently angled sufficiently to the right and the left to scan out to the Sylvian fissures and insulae on both sides (see Part II). Because the lateral ventricles fan out posteriorly, the transducer should be positioned slightly slanting, with the posterior part of the transducer slightly more lateral than the anterior part. The second and fourth parasagittal planes enable visualisation of the lateral ventricles over their entire length (see Fig. 3.5 and Part II). The third and fifth parasagittal planes show the insulae (see Part II).

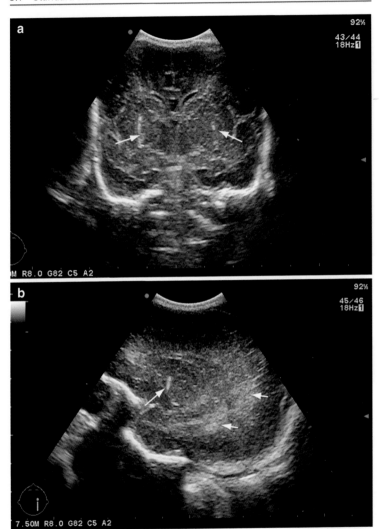

Fig. 3.2 (**a, b**) Ultrasound scan in a preterm infant, showing lenticulostriate vasculopathy (*arrows*), seen in two image directions. (**a**) Coronal scan at the level of the frontal horns of the lateral ventricles. (**b**) Parasagittal scan, also showing inhomogeneous echogenicity of the periventricular white matter (*short arrows*)

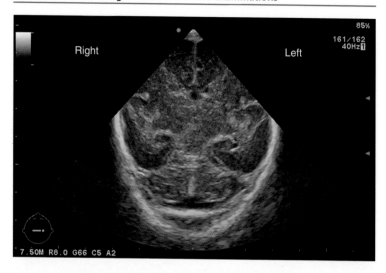

Fig. 3.3 Coronal ultrasound scan in a very preterm infant at the level of the bodies of the lateral ventricles. If the marker on the transducer is positioned in the right corner of the anterior fontanel (*see* Figs. 2.1, 2.2a and 3.1), the right side of the brain is projected on the left side of the image, and vice versa

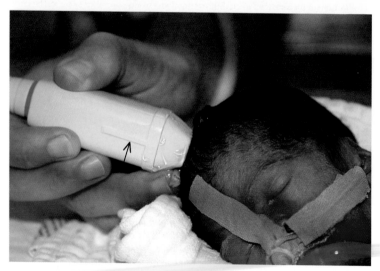

Fig. 3.4 Probe positioning for obtaining sagittal planes. *Arrow* indicates marker

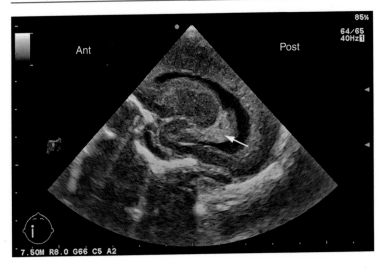

Fig. 3.5 Parasagittal ultrasound scan in a very preterm infant (GA 25 weeks) through the left lateral ventricle. If the marker on the transducer is pointing towards the baby's nose (see Fig. 3.4), the anterior part of the brain will be projected on the left of the image and the posterior part on the right. Image shows large, bulky choroid plexus (*arrow*) and wide occipital horn of the lateral ventricle, both phenomena being normal for this age. The body marker at the bottom of the image indicates that the left side of the brain is depicted

When scanning in the sagittal planes, it is important to mark which side of the brain is being scanned. This can either be done using the body marker application or by an annotation (see Figs. 3.5 and 3.6).

3.2   Supplemental Acoustic Windows

If only the anterior fontanel is used as an acoustic window, brain structures further away from this fontanel cannot be visualised with high-frequency transducers. Lower frequencies enable deeper penetration (see Fig. 2.5), but detailed information is lost. Better visualisation can be obtained using acoustic windows closer to these structures, thus allowing the use of higher-frequency, high-resolution transducers and visualisation from different angles (Fig. 3.7).

Using these supplemental acoustic windows for cUS examinations requires additional skills, practice and anatomical knowledge. The views thus obtained

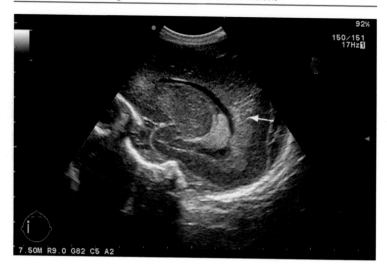

Fig. 3.6 Parasagittal ultrasound scan in a very preterm infant (GA 28 weeks) through the left lateral ventricle, as is shown by the body marker. Image shows bulky choroid plexus (normal for this age) and mildly increased echogenicity of the parietal periventricular white matter (*arrow*)

and the anatomical structures visualised are presented in Part II. In order to avoid excessive manipulation of the infant, it is recommended to use only those acoustic windows that are easily accessible (i.e. if the infant is positioned on its left side, only the right-sided windows are used, and vice versa). The examination can be continued when the infant's position is changed.

Indications for cUS using supplemental windows are presented in Appendix 3.1.

3.2.1   Posterior Fontanel

The posterior fontanel, located between the parietal and occipital bones (see Fig. 3.7), enables a good view of the occipital and temporal horns of the lateral ventricles, the occipital and temporal parenchyma, and the posterior fossa structures. Using this fontanel, scanning can be done in coronal and sagittal planes. The posterior fontanel is palpated and the transducer

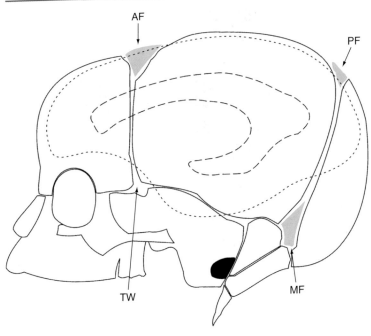

Fig. 3.7 The acoustic windows. *AF* anterior fontanel, *PF* posterior fontanel, *MF* mastoid (or postero-lateral) fontanel, *TW* temporal window

placed in the middle of the fontanel, with the marker in the horizontal position to obtain a coronal plane and in the vertical position to obtain a sagittal plane (Fig. 3.8). Scanning through the posterior fontanel enables more accurate detection of haemorrhage in the occipital horns of the lateral ventricles, injury to the occipital and temporal lobes, cerebellar haemorrhage, and posterior fossa malformations (Figs. 3.9–3.11).

3.2.2   Temporal Windows

Good transverse views of the brain stem can be obtained through the temporal window. The transducer is placed above the ear, approximately 1 cm above and anterior to the external auditory meatus, with the marker

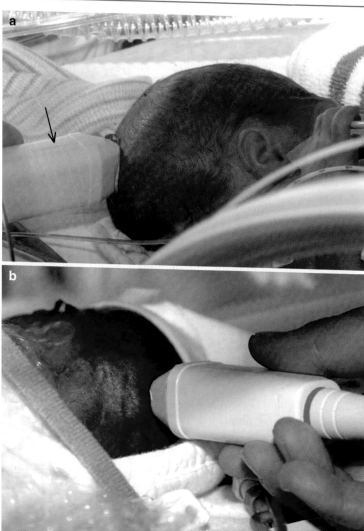

Fig. 3.8 (**a**, **b**) Posterior fontanel. (**a**) Probe positioning for coronal scan using the posterior fontanel as an acoustic window (*arrow* indicates marker). (**b**) Probe positioning for parasagittal scan using the posterior fontanel as an acoustic window. The marker (not shown here) is on the top of the probe, pointing towards the cranium

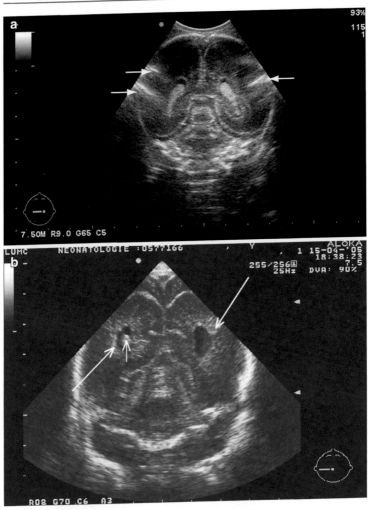

Fig. 3.9 (**a–c**) Coronal ultrasound scans obtained through the posterior fontanel in very preterm infants. (**a**) Artefacts (*arrows*) caused by suboptimal contact between transducer and skull. (**b**) Increased echogenicity in the occipital white matter (*arrows*) and a blood clot in the occipital horn of the right lateral ventricle (*short arrow*). (**c**) Intraventricular haemorrhage with blood clots in the occipital horn of the left lateral ventricle (*arrows*). (Suboptimal image quality, due to insufficient contact between transducer and skull)

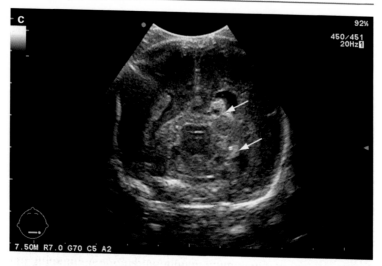

Fig. 3.9 (continued)

in a horizontal position. The transducer position is subsequently adjusted until the brain stem is visualised (Fig. 3.12). The image quality in this view depends on the bony thickness. Scanning through the temporal window allows Doppler flow measurements in the circle of Willis and detection of brain stem and cerebellar haemorrhages (Fig. 3.13).

3.2.3   Mastoid Fontanels

The mastoid fontanels are located at the junction of the temporal, occipital, and posterior parietal bones (see Fig. 3.7). These windows allow visualisation of the posterior fossa and the midbrain in two planes (Fig. 3.14), thus enabling detection of congenital anomalies and haemorrhages in these areas, in particular cerebellar haemorrhages (Fig. 3.15) and dilatation of the third and fourth ventricles. In our experience also ischaemic cerebellar injury can be detected using the mastoid fontanels (Fig. 3.16).

After the auricle is gently bent forward, the transducer is placed behind the ear, just above the tragus, and subsequently moved until a good view of the posterior fossa is obtained. If the transducer is positioned with the

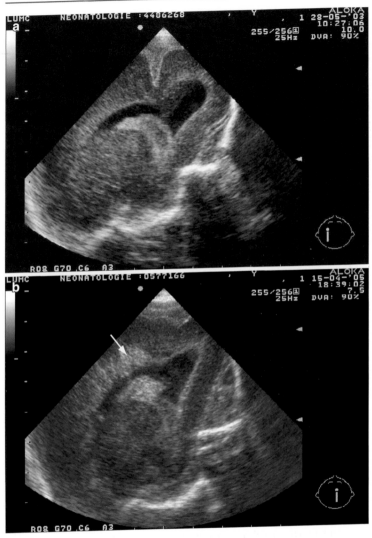

Fig. 3.10 (**a, b**) Parasagittal ultrasound scans obtained through the posterior fontanel in a very preterm infant. (**a**) Normal. (**b**) Increased echogenicity in the periventricular white matter (*arrow*) (same patient as in Fig. 3.9b)

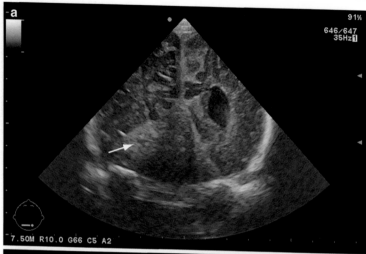

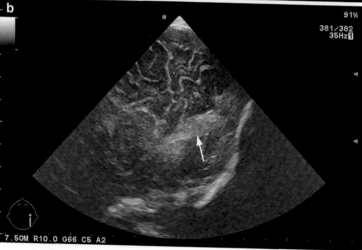

Fig 3.11 (**a**, **b**) Coronal (**a**) and parasagittal (**b**) cUS scans obtained through the posterior fontanel in a full-term neonate who presented with convulsions on the 2nd of life. cUS shows echodensity in the right temporal lobe (*arrows*) suggesting haemorrhage, which was confirmed by MRI. Also note the dilatation of the left occipital horn

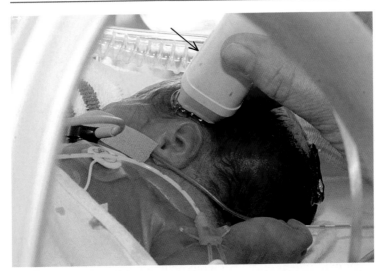

Fig. 3.12 Temporal window. Probe positioning for cUS using temporal window, providing transverse views (*arrow* indicates marker)

marker in a vertical direction, a coronal plane is obtained. If the marker is in a horizontal position, a transverse view is obtained (see Fig. 3.14).

3.3 Doppler Flow Measurements

(Colour) Doppler ultrasonography can be applied to study cerebral haemo-dynamics. Blood flow velocity can be measured in the major cerebral arter-ies and their branches and in the basilar and internal carotid arteries (see Fig. 3.13b) and the large veins (i.e. internal cerebral veins, vein of Galen, superior sagittal, straight and transverse sinus). Doppler flow measurements may help to distinguish between vascular structures and non-vascular lesions. Blood flow velocities in the major cerebral arteries can be of prognostic significance in infants with hypoxic-ischaemic brain injury.

A detailed overview of the role of cerebral Doppler imaging is provided in the book by Couture and Veyrac 2001.

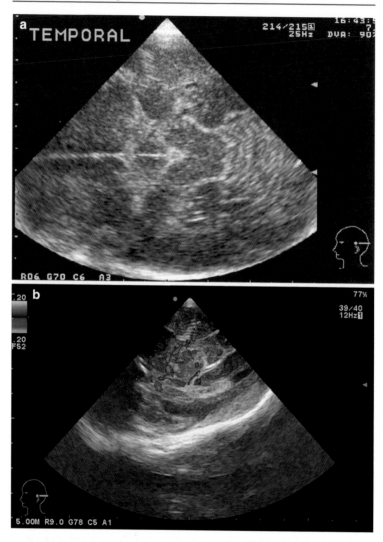

Fig. 3.13 (**a**, **b**) Temporal window. (**a**) Normal transverse view of brain stem and upper cerebellum, obtained through temporal window. (**b**) Transverse view of brain stem showing circle of Willis, using colour Doppler

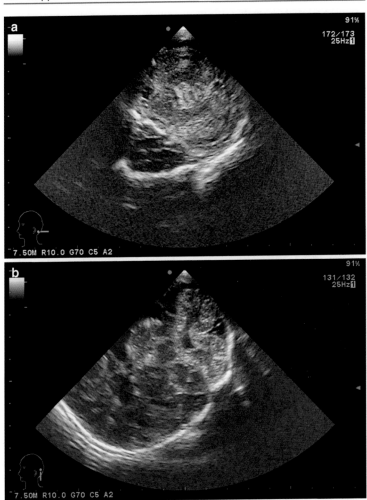

Fig. 3.14 (**a, b**) cUS through the left mastoid fontanel in a near-term baby (gestational age 36 weeks). (**a**) Axial view and (**b**) coronal view, showing a normal cerebellum. Note the normal difference in echogenicity between the hemisphere closest to the transducer and the hemisphere farthest from the transducer

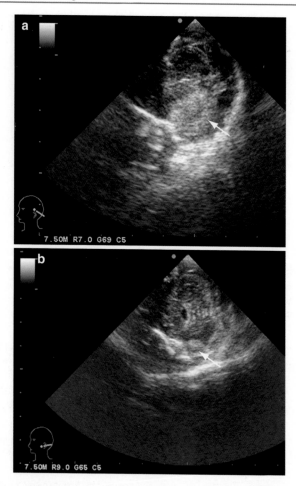

Fig. 3.15 (**a, b**) cUS through the left mastoid fontanel in very preterm neonates. (**a**) Oblique axial view, showing large irregular echodensity in the right cerebellar hemisphere (*arrow*), diagnosed as cerebellar haemorrhage (confirmed by MRI). (**b**) Oblique axial view, showing small echodensity in the right cerebellar hemisphere (*arrow*), diagnosed as small cerebellar haemorrhage (confirmed by MRI)

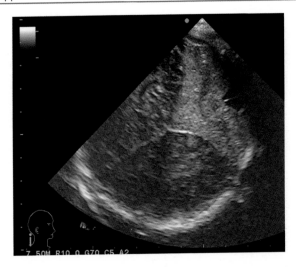

Fig. 3.16 cUS through the right mastoid fontanel in full-term newborn with hypoxic-ischaemic encephalopathy, showing diffusely increased echogenicity of the cerebellar hemispheres, with loss of the normal architecture. MRI confirmed hypoxic-ischaemic cerebellar injury

Standard cUS procedure	Supplemental acoustic windows
• Anterior fontanel = acoustic window (supratentorial structures) • Scan whole brain from frontal to occipital and right to left • Record at least six standard coronal and five standard (para)-sagittal planes • Record (suspected) abnormalities in two planes	• Posterior fontanel (occipital and temporal parenchyma, occipital and temporal horns, posterior fossa) • Temporal windows (midbrain, circle of Willis, flow measurements) • Mastoid fontanels (midbrain, posterior fossa, ventricular system)

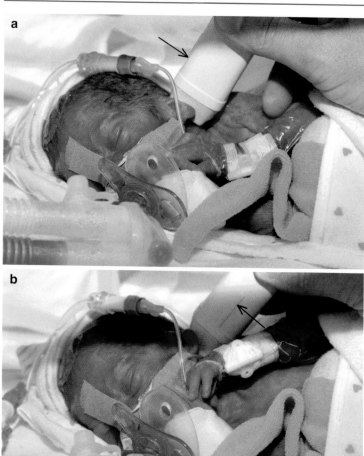

Fig. 3.17 (**a**, **b**) Mastoid fontanel. (**a**) Probe position for coronal view using the mastoid fontanel as an acoustic window. (**b**) Probe position for transverse view using the mastoid fontanel as an acoustic window. *Arrows* indicate marker on probe

Appendix 3.1: Indications for Scanning Through Supplemental Windows

- Preterm, gestational age (GA) < 30 weeks, around third day (cerebellar haemorrhage?)
- Preterm, complicated medical course with circulatory and/or respiratory instability
- Peri- and intraventricular haemorrhage (haemorrhage in occipital horns and/or fourth ventricle? Cerebellar haemorrhage?)
- Suspected posterior fossa haemorrhage on standard cUS
- (Antenatally) suspected posterior fossa abnormalities
- Congenital malformations
- Ventricular dilatation of unknown cause
- (Suspected) metabolic disease
- Hypoxic-ischaemic brain injury in the (near) term neonate
- Unexplained neurological symptoms

Reference

Couture A, Veyrac C (2001) Transfontanellar Doppler imaging in neonates, 1st edn. Springer, Berlin

Further Reading

Correa F et al (2004) Posterior fontanelle sonography: an acoustic window into the neonatal brain. AJNR Am J Neuroradiol 25:1274–1282

Couture A et al (2001) Advanced cranial ultrasound: transfontanellar Doppler imaging in neonates. Eur Radiol 11:2399–2410

Di Salvo DN (2001) A new view of the neonatal brain: clinical utility of supplemental neurologic US imaging windows. Radiographics 21:943–955

Steggerda SJ et al (2009a) Neonatal cranial ultrasonography: how to optimize its performance. Early Hum Dev 85:93–99

Steggerda SJ et al (2009b) Cerebellar injury in preterm infants: incidence and findings on ultrasound and MRI. Radiology 252:190–199

Taylor GA (1992) Intracranial venous system in the newborn: evaluation of normal anatomy and flow characteristics with color Doppler US. Radiology 183:449–452

4.1   Assessing Cranial Ultrasound Examinations

When performing and assessing cUS examinations, the *anatomy* (see Part II) and *maturation* (see Part I Chap. 8) of the brain are evaluated, and signs of *pathology*, whether congenital or acquired, are sought. In general, anomalies should be visualised in at least two different planes (see Fig. 3.2). An overview of brain pathology as can be visualised by cUS is provided in the *Atlas on Cranial Ultrasonography* by Govaert and De Vries 2010.

4.1.1   A Systematic Approach to Detect Cerebral Pathology

While looking for anomalies, a systematic approach is recommended. The following can be used as a guideline:

- Are the *anatomical* structures distinguishable, and do they appear normal? (See Part II; Fig. 4.1)
- Does the *maturation* of the brain (cortical folding) appear appropriate for GA? (See Chap. 8; Fig. 4.2 see Fig. 4.1a)
- Is there a normal distinction between the cortex and the white matter? (Fig. 4.3)
- Is the echogenicity of the cortical grey matter normal? (Fig. 4.4)
- Is the echogenicity of the periventricular and subcortical white matter normal and homogeneous? (Fig. 4.5)

G. Meijler, *Neonatal Cranial Ultrasonography*,
DOI 10.1007/978-3-642-21320-5_4,
© Springer-Verlag Berlin Heidelberg 2012

- Is there normal echogenicity and homogeneity of the thalami and basal ganglia? (Fig. 4.6)
- Do the size, width, lining and echogenicity of the ventricular system appear normal? (Figs. 4.7 and 4.8)
- In the case of ventricular enlargement, the lateral ventricles are measured according to standard guidelines. (Fig. 4.8) (Levene 1981; Davies et al. 2000; Brouwer et al. 2011; see also Appendix 4.1 and Figs. 4.11–4.14)
- Are the widths of the subarachnoid spaces appropriate for age? (Fig. 4.9)
- Is there a midline shift? (Fig. 4.10)

Image assessment
<ul><li>Anatomy</li><li>Maturation</li><li>Distinction between cortex/white matter</li><li>Echogenicity of cortex</li><li>Echogenicity/homogeneity of white matter</li><li>Echogenicity/homogeneity of deep grey matter</li><li>Ventricular system: size, lining, echogenicity; If dilated: perform serial measurements</li><li>Width of subarachnoid spaces</li><li>Midline shift</li></ul>

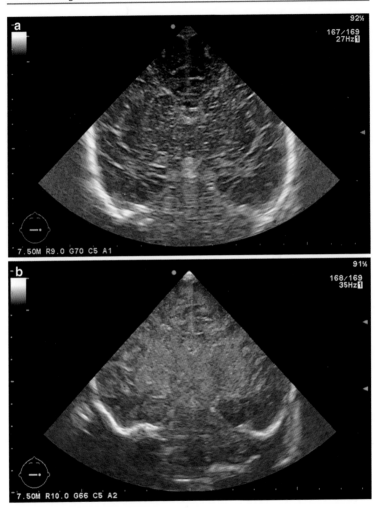

Fig. 4.1 (**a, b**) Coronal ultrasound scans obtained in full-term neonates at the level of the frontal horns of the lateral ventricles. (**a**) Normal image. (**b**) Loss of normal architecture and diffusely increased echogenicity in a neonate with severe hypoxic-ischaemic brain injury

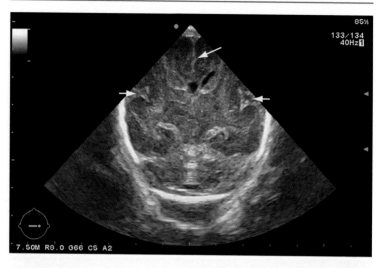

Fig. 4.2 Coronal ultrasound scan at the level of the frontal horns of the lateral ventricles in a very preterm infant (GA 25 + 3 weeks), showing smooth interhemispheric fissure (*arrow*) and wide open Sylvian fissures (*short arrows*). Brain maturation appropriate for GA. Also showing asymmetry of the lateral ventricles, being a normal finding in (preterm) neonates. Compare image with (Fig. 4.1a)

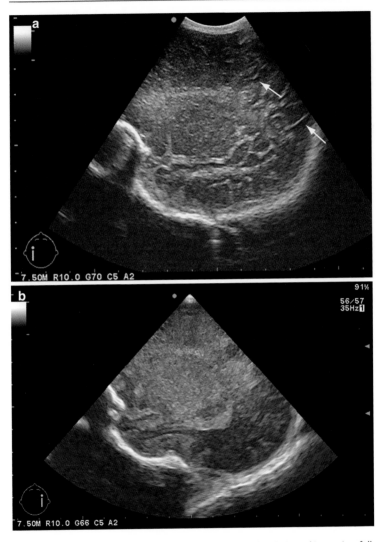

Fig. 4.3 (**a**, **b**) Parasagittal ultrasound scan through the insula. (**a**) Normal image in a full-term neonate, showing normal hypo-echogenic cortex (*arrows*) and distinction between cortex and white matter. (**b**) Loss of normal grey–white matter differentiation with blurring of the cortex in a full-term neonate with hypoxic-ischaemic brain injury

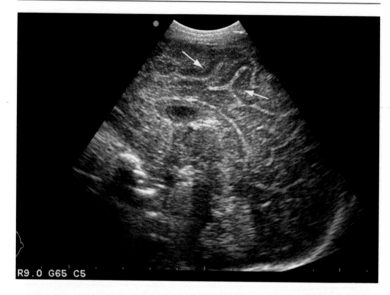

Fig. 4.4 Midsagittal ultrasound scan in a full-term baby with hypoxic-ischaemic brain injury, showing a widened hypo-echogenic cortex (*arrows*), indicating cortical injury

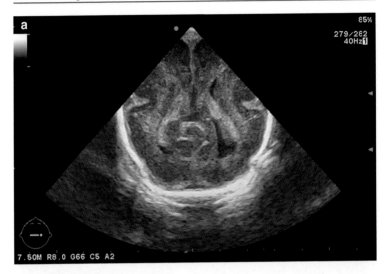

Fig. 4.5 (**a**, **b**) Preterm infant (GA 25 + 3 weeks) with normal echogenicity of the periventricular white matter, being less than that of the choroid plexus. (**a**) Coronal view through the trigone of the lateral ventricles. (**b**) Parasagittal view. (**c**) Preterm infant (GA 32 weeks), coronal cUS through the parieto-occipital lobes, showing homogeneously increased echogenicity of the parietal periventricular white matter (*arrows*): periventricular echodensity (PVE) or "flaring." (**d**, **e**) cUS scan in preterm infant (GA 31 + 3 weeks), showing inhomogeneously increased echogenicity of the periventricular white matter (*arrows*), indicating white matter injury (**d**) coronal scan through the parieto-occipital lobes, (**e**) parasagittal scan through the right lateral ventricle. (**f**) Parasagittal CUS scan in preterm infant (GA 36 weeks) with enterovirus encephalitis, showing inhomogeneously increased echogenicity of the parietal white matter, extending into the subcortical white matter (*arrows*)

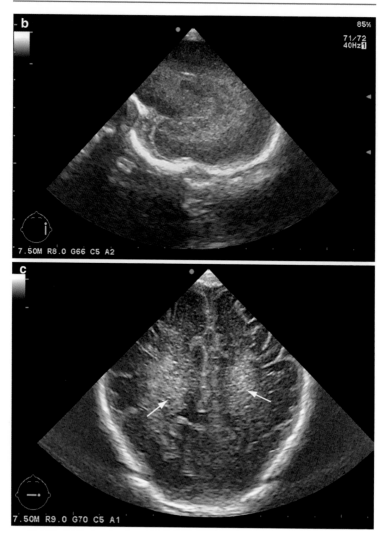

Fig. 4.5 (continued)

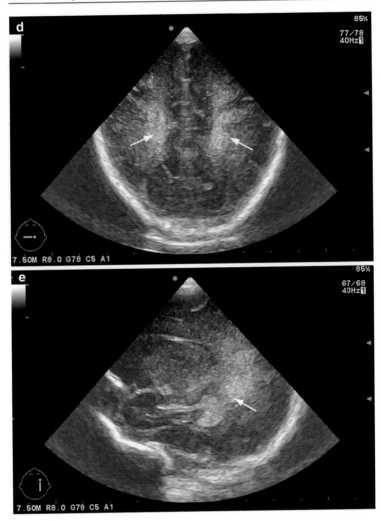

Fig. 4.5 (continued)

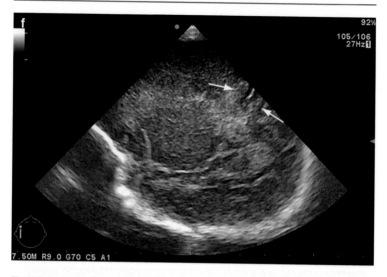

Fig. 4.5 (continued)

Fig. 4.6 (**a**, **b**) cUS scan in preterm infant (GA 25 + 3 weeks), showing subtle, diffuse echoge-nicity of the basal ganglia (*arrows*). (**a**) Coronal view through the frontal horns of the lateral ventricles. (**b**) Parasagittal view. This is a normal finding in very preterm neonates until term equivalent age. Also showing wide occipital horn of the lateral ventricle, asymmetry of the lateral ventricles and bulky choroid plexus, all being normal findings at this age. (**c**, **d**) cUS scan in full-term neonate with hypoxic-ischaemic brain injury, showing increased echogenic-ity in the basal ganglia and thalami (*arrows*), indicating deep grey matter injury in (near) term neonates. (**c**) Coronal view through the frontal horns of the lateral ventricles. (**d**) Parasagittal view, also showing widened hypo-echogenic cortex (*short arrow*), indicating cortical injury. (**e**) cUS scan in a preterm neonate (GA 30 weeks) parasagittal view showing localized echodensity in the left thalamic region (*arrow*), presenting infarction

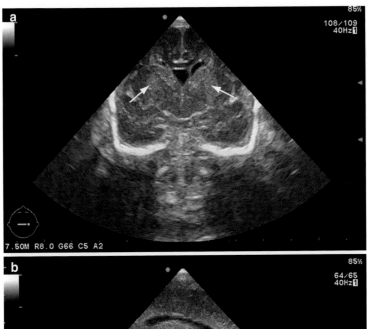

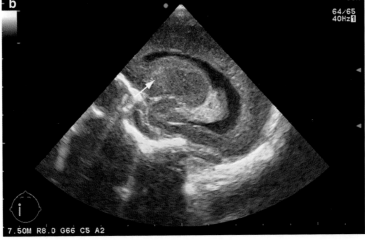

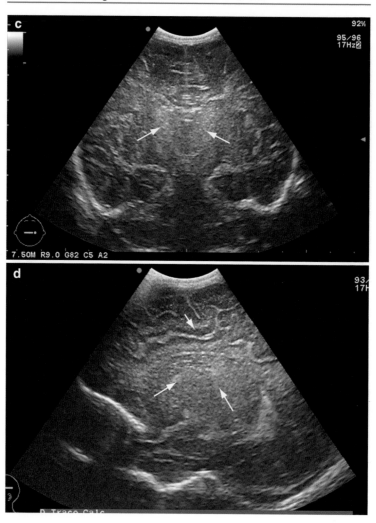

Fig. 4.6 (continued)

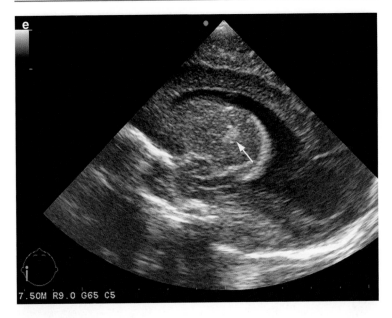

Fig. 4.6 (continued)

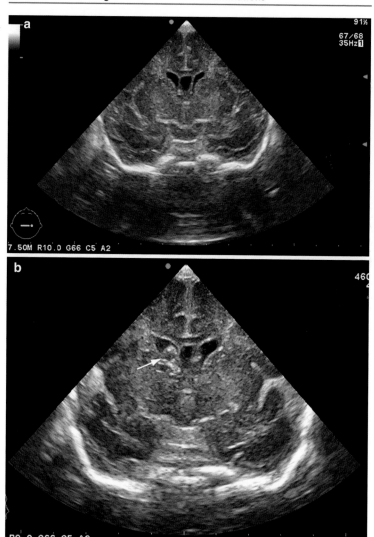

Fig. 4.7 (**a–c**) Coronal cUS scans at the level of the frontal horns of the lateral ventricles in a preterm infant (GA 32 weeks), showing in (**a**) normal lateral ventricles without haemorrhage on first day of life. In (**b**) 3 days later: intraventricular haemorrhage with blood clot in the right lateral ventricle (*arrow*) and (**c**) subsequent dilatation of the lateral ventricles with echogenic ventricular lining (*arrowhead*) and strand in left frontal horn

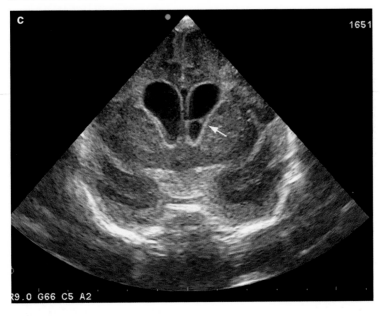

Fig. 4.7 (continued)

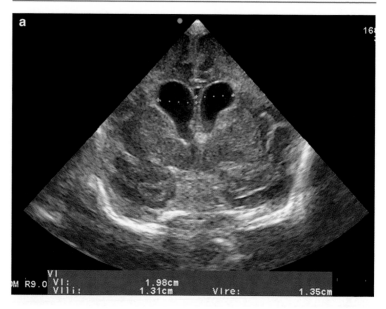

Fig. 4.8 (**a, b**) Same preterm infant as Fig. 4.7. (**a, b**) Coronal cUS scans at the level of the frontal horns of the ventricles and the foramen of Monro: (**a**) measurement of ventricular index according to Levene. (**b**) Measurement of the anterior horn width according to Davies. (**c**) Parasagittal scan through the left lateral ventricle: measurement of the thalamo-occipital distance according to Davies

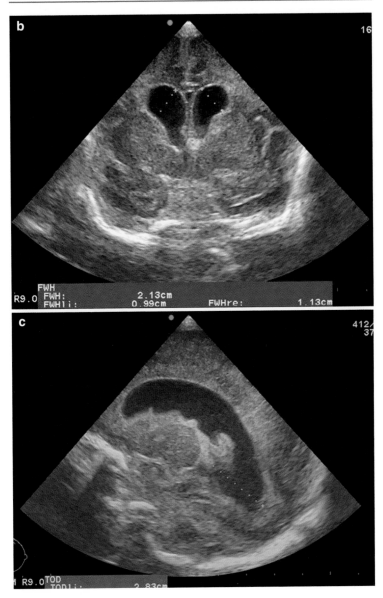

Fig. 4.8 (continued)

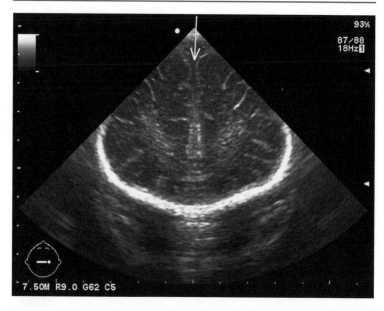

Fig. 4.9 Coronal cUS scan at the level of the frontal lobes in a very preterm infant scanned at term age, showing wide subarachnoid space (*arrow*)

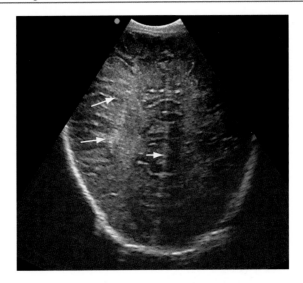

Fig. 4.10 Coronal cUS scan at the level of the parieto-occipital lobes in a full-term neonate presenting with convulsions. cUS shows asymmetric echogenicity of the right hemisphere (*arrows*), suggestive of middle cerebral artery infarction (confirmed by MRI). Midline shift towards the left, due to swelling of the right hemisphere (*short arrow*)

Fig. 4.11 (a–c) Reference curves for the (**a**) ventricular index, (**b**) anterior horn width, and (**c**) thalamo-occipital distance, related to postmenstrual age at scanning. Presented are the estimated means and 95% reference intervals fitted to the ventricular measurements (Adapted from Brouwer MJ et al. 2012) (see also Appendix 4.1)

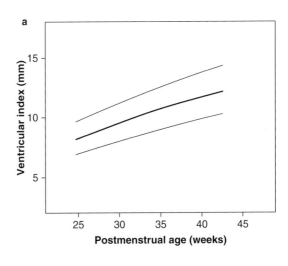

Fig. 4.11 (continued)

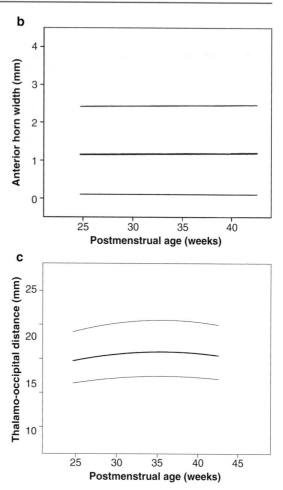

Appendix 4.1: Measurement of the Lateral Ventricles

- *Ventricular index* (VI): the distance between the falx and the lateral wall of the anterior horn (coronal plane) (Levene 1981)
- *Anterior horn width* (AHW): the diagonal width of the anterior horn measured at its widest point (coronal plane) (Davies et al. 2000)
- *Thalamo-occipital distance* (TOD): the distance between the thalamus and the outer border of the occipital horn (parasagittal plane) (Davies et al. 2000)

In the third coronal plane (at the level of the interventricular foramina of Monro), the ventricular width is measured as the largest distance in millimetres between the frontal horns. This number, if divided by 2, results in the VI according to Levene. New reference values are available (Brouwer et al. 2012) (Fig. 4.11; see also Fig. 4.8a).

The width of the anterior horn of the lateral ventricles (AHW) is measured in the third coronal plane (at the level of the interventricular foramina of Monro). The width is measured on each side as the distance between the medial wall and the floor of the lateral ventricle at the widest point. New reference values are available (Brouwer et al. 2012) (Figs. 4.11 and 4.12, see also Fig. 4.8b).

In the second and fourth parasagittal planes, the TOD is measured on each side as the distance between the outermost point of the thalamus at its junction with the choroid plexus and the outermost part of the occipital horn. New reference values are available. (Brouwer et al. 2012) (Fig. 4.11; see also Fig.4.8c)

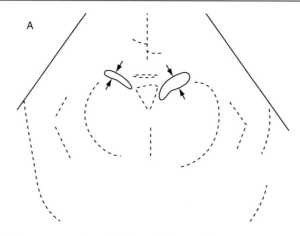

Fig. 4.12 Measurement of anterior horn width, according to Davies et al. 2000 (see also Appendix 4.1). Reproduced with permission from BMJ Publishing Group

References

Brouwer MJ et al (2012) New reference values for the neonatal cerebral ventricles. Radiology 262(1):224–233. Epub 2011

Davies MW et al (2000) Reference ranges for the linear dimensions of the intracranial ventricles in preterm neonates. Arch Dis Child Fetal Neonatal Ed 82:F218–F223

Govaert P, De Vries LS (2010) An atlas of neonatal brain sonography, 2nd edn. MacKeith Press, Cambridge

Levene MI (1981) Measurement of the growth of the lateral ventricles in preterm infants with real-time ultrasound. Arch Dis Child 56:900–904

Further Reading

Enriquez G et al (2003) Potential pitfalls in cranial sonography. Pediatr Radiol 33(2):110–117

Leijser LM et al (2010) Is sequential cranial ultrasound reliable for detection of white matter injury in very preterm infants? Neuroradiology 52(5):397–406

Van Wezel-Meijler G et al (2011) Diffuse hyperechogenicity of the basal ganglia and thalami in preterm infants: a physiological finding? Radiology 258(3):944–950

5.1 Timing of Ultrasound Examinations

To obtain optimal information from cUS serial, carefully timed examinations are essential, both in preterm and sick full-term infants. If timing is not optimally chosen, time intervals between cUS examinations are too long, or cUS examinations are discontinued too early, important information and/or injury may be overlooked. On the other hand, if the quality of cUS is good, timing is well chosen, proper transducers are used, and, in the case of preterm birth, serial examinations are continued until term equivalent age, most abnormalities will be detected. Serial cUS examinations are not only essential for accurate and reliable detection of brain damage, but they also enable assessment of brain growth and maturation, timing of injury and the evolution of lesions.

5.1.1 Cranial Ultrasound Screening

In neonatal units, it is useful to apply general guidelines for cUS examinations (see Chaps. 3 and 4) and a cUS screening protocol. Scanning protocols vary considerably between neonatal units. In Appendix 5.1, a useful screening protocol is presented. It is based on the results of recent neuroimaging studies, examining the performance of cUS and can be applied to all neonates admitted to a neonatal unit, including preterm neonates, sick full-term neonates, neonates with neurological symptoms and neonates with congenital malformations. It calls for at least one cUS examination, regardless of GA, diagnosis or medical course, and serial cUS examinations for preterm and sick full-term neonates.

G. Meijler, *Neonatal Cranial Ultrasonography*,
DOI 10.1007/978-3-642-21320-5_5,
© Springer-Verlag Berlin Heidelberg 2012

This screening protocol is based on the following:

- A first cUS examination soon after birth will give information on congenital anomalies of the brain, congenital infections, some inborn errors of metabolism, traumatic brain injury and the antenatal onset of lesions. It can also serve as a baseline and comparison for the following cUS examinations.
- Haemorrhagic lesions usually become visible within hours of the incident.
- Most haemorrhagic lesions in newborn infants develop around birth.
- More than 90% of germinal matrix- intraventricular haemorrhages (GMH-IVH) develop within the first 3 days of birth.
- Progression of an initial GMH-IVH usually occurs within the first week.
- Thus, a first cUS examination performed soon after birth (within 24 h) and a second examination performed around the third day of life will enable detection of congenital anomalies, antenatally acquired lesions and most haemorrhagic lesions. By performing a third scan around the seventh day, almost all haemorrhages will be detected and their maximum extent identified alinea.
- It takes a variable period of time (hours to days) before ischaemic lesions become visible.
- The first stages of hypoxic-ischaemic brain injury may evolve over a variable period of time (hours to weeks).

Fig. 5.1 (**a–f**) (**a**) Coronal cUS scan at the level of the frontal lobes in a preterm infant (GA 27 weeks), showing symmetrical, bilateral echogenicity in the frontal white matter ("frontal echodensities") (*arrows*), which is a normal finding in preterm infants (van Wezel-Meijler et al. 1998). (**b**) These normal frontal echodensities should not be confused with pathological periventricular echodensities (PVE) (*arrows*): Coronal cUS scan at the level of the frontal lobes in a very preterm infant, showing asymmetric, inhomogeneous periventricular echodensities in the frontal white matter. (**c**) Coronal cUS scan at the level of the frontal horns in a very preterm infant (GA 28 + 2 weeks), showing subtle echogenicity in the basal ganglia (*arrows*). (**d**) This normal phenomenon at this age (van Wezel-Meijler et al. 2011a) should not be confused with abnormally increased echogenicity in the same region (preterm neonate, GA 30 weeks): asymmetric, inhomogeneous echogenicity in the basal ganglia (*arrows*). (**e**) Coronal cUS scan in very preterm infant (GA 25 + 3 weeks), showing echogenicity in the parietal region, adjacent to the lateral ventricles (*arrow*). This normal phenomenon at this age (Boxma et al. 2005) should not be confused with pathological PVE in the same region: (**f**) cUS scan in preterm infant, showing inhomogeneous, echogenicity in the right parietal area (*arrow*). These PVE gradually became more intense and widespread, and eventually evolved into cystic lesions

- Especially in preterm infants, the first stages and the milder spectrum of hypoxic-ischaemic brain injury may be hard to distinguish from normal (maturational) phenomena occurring in the immature brain (*Fig. 5.1*).

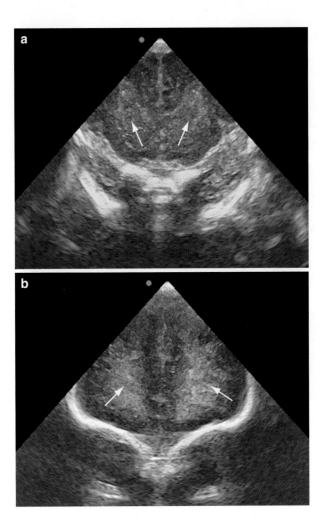

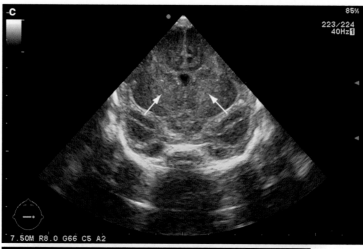

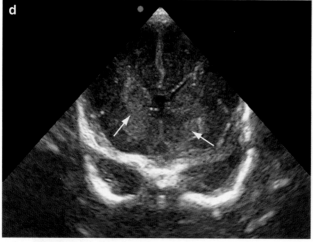

Fig. 5.1 (continued)

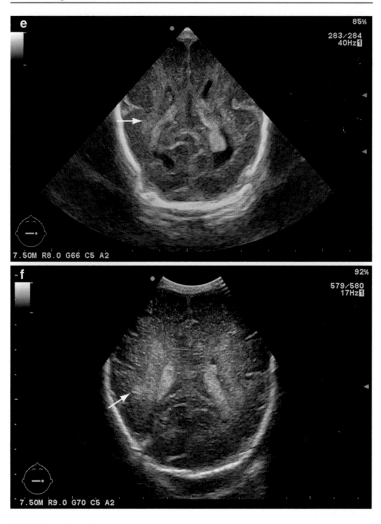

Fig. 5.1 (continued)

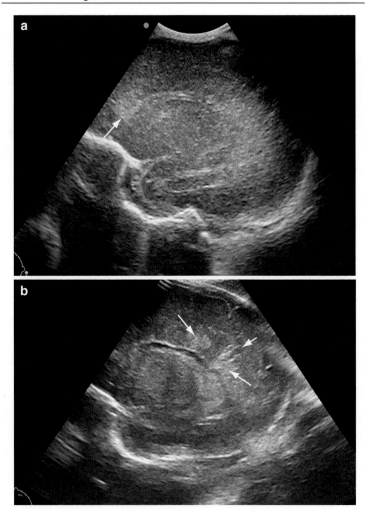

Fig. 5.2 (**a**) Parasagittal cUS in a very preterm infant (GA 29 weeks, same infant as *Fig. 5.1f*), initially showing normal echogenicity of the periventricular white matter. Also showing physiological frontal echodensity (*arrow*). (**b**) This infant had a complicated respiratory course and septicemia and later developed serious periventricular leukomalacia: parasagittal cUS scan 2 weeks later showing inhomogeneous echodensities (*arrows*) with precystic lesions (*short arrow*) in the fronto-parietal region

An overview on how to distinguish normal, physiological periventricular echodensities (PVE) in the white matter from pathological echodensities is given in Appendix 5.2.

- In preterm infants, ischaemic lesions may develop throughout the neonatal period, related to postnatal events (*Fig. 5.2*).
- Diffuse or subtle white matter injury, frequently encountered in very preterm neonates, is not well detected with cUS. Subtle white matter injury may be of importance for neurodevelopmental outcome and is reliably evaluated using MRI.

Thus:

- A cUS examination performed on the first day of life and repeated during the first week enables detection of the acute stages of perinatal hypoxic-ischaemic brain injury.
- Sequential cUS examinations are needed to assess the evolution of ischaemic lesions and to distinguish (mild) pathology from normal (maturational) phenomena.
- In preterm infants, sequential cUS examinations throughout the neonatal period are necessary to follow brain growth and development and to detect later onset of (ischaemic) injury.
- In very preterm infants, MRI is needed for reliable diagnosis of white matter injury.

For infants who were born prematurely and are later transferred from the referral centre to a local hospital, arrangements need to be made for continuation of cUS examinations. If local facilities are insufficient, it is recommended that cUS examinations be performed at regular intervals at the neonatal centre.

5.2   Cranial Ultrasonography at Term Corrected Age

In infants born very prematurely (GA < 32 weeks) and/or with very low birth weight (< 1,500 g), it is recommended that cUS be performed around term equivalent age (TEA), preferably at the neonatal centre. This term examination is done to see the later stages of (ischaemic) brain injury, to detect new lesions that may have developed after discharge *(see Fig. 5.2)*, and to evaluate brain growth and development *(see Fig. 4.9)*. cUS examinations performed around TEA may show:

- Cysts in regression, within the spectrum of cystic periventricular leukomalacia (PVL) (see Chap. 6)
- Cysts within the spectrum of late onset cystic-PVL
- Ex-vacuo ventricular dilatation, following white matter injury, often associated with increased width of the subarachnoid space and widening of the interhemispheric fissure
- Post haemorrhagic ventricular dilatation (PHVD) following a germinal matrix-intraventricular haemorrhage (GMH-IVH) (see Chap. 6)
- Cystic phase of periventricular haemorrhagic infarction (PVHI) (see Chap. 6)
- Cystic phase of focal arterial infarction

In very preterm infants in whom MRI is performed around TEA, a term cUS examination will not contribute to the detection of white matter injury, but it may detect lesions that are generally better depicted with cUS than with MRI, including germinolytic cysts, lenticulostriate vasculopathy and calcifications (Leijser et al. 2009a, van Wezel-Meijler 2011b).

5.3   Adaptations of Ultrasound Examinations, Depending on Diagnosis

When using a cUS screening protocol, it is important to realise that routine screening is suitable for neonates without neurological symptoms or brain pathology and for neonates with stable brain abnormalities (such as congenital anomalies or stabilised, acquired lesions). In cases of (suspected) cUS and/or neurological abnormalities, the intensity and frequency of cUS examinations may need to be increased, depending on the clinical picture and the lesion(s) (Appendix 5.1). This can vary between one or two cUS examinations a week in non-progressive cases and several cUS examinations a day in unstable cases (such as IVH with PHVD, severe hypoxic-ischaemic encephalopathy, complicated meningitis, and brain infections).

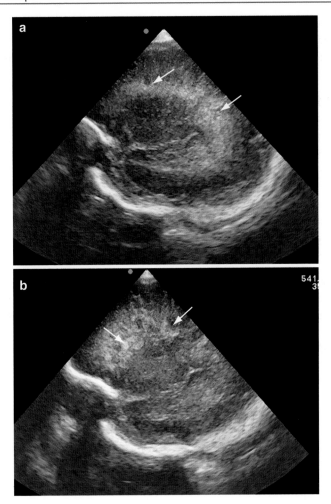

Fig. 5.3 (**a–c**) Parasagittal ultrasound scans in a preterm infant (GA 31 weeks). (**a**) Initially showing periventricular echodensities (*arrows*) in the fronto-parietal region. (**b**) Later evolving into more echogenic and inhomogeneous echodensities (*arrows*) and (**c**) cystic lesions, which developed only after several weeks

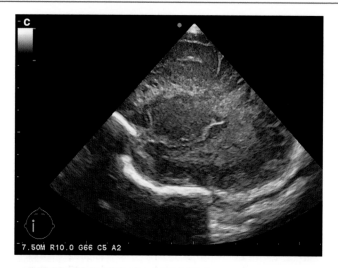

Fig. 5.3 (continued)

If complications occur after GMH-IVH (progression of the haemorrhage, PHVD, and/or PVHI) (see Chap. 6), it is recommended that the frequency of cUS examinations be intensified and, in the case of ventricular dilatation, the lateral ventricles be measured on a regular basis until stabilisation has occurred (see Chaps. 4 and 6).

It is also important to realise that the end stages of hypoxic-ischaemic brain damage may not become visible until a variable period of time, often several weeks to months after the event, and that the early stages may seem mild or subtle (*Figs. 5.3 and 5.4*, see Chap. 6). In cases of (suspected) ischaemic injury, even if apparently mild, it is therefore advisable to intensify cUS examinations until normalisation or stabilisation of abnormalities has occurred.

Meningitis and brain infections can have a very rapid, fulminant course and should therefore be intensively monitored by repetitive cUS *(Fig. 5.5)*.

It needs to be emphasised once more that if the timing of cUS is not optimal the first stages of injury may be missed, milder and/or diffuse injury overlooked, and complications of haemorrhages or infections detected late or not at all. In addition, if cUS examinations are discontinued too early (the severe end stages of) injury may remain undetected.

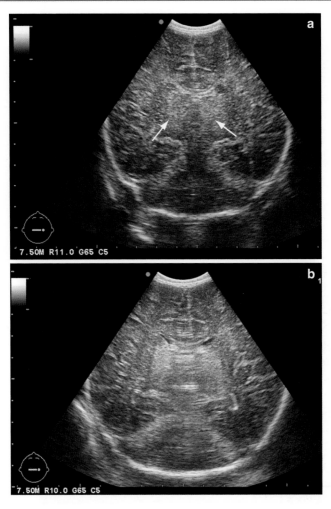

Fig. 5.4 (**a** and **b**) Coronal ultrasound scan in a full-term neonate, born asphyxiated. (**a**) First scan, performed several hours after birth, showing echogenicity in the thalami (*arrows*). (**b**) A few days later the echogenicity is more seriously increased and the brain anatomy is shown in less detail. Compare with normal image *(Fig. 4.1a)*

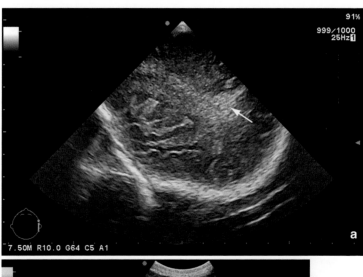

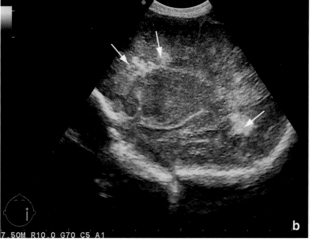

Fig. 5.5 Parasagittal ultrasound scans (**a**) and (**b**) in a preterm infant (GA 36 weeks) with enterovirus encephalitis. This infant initially had normal cUS findings, but developed white matter injury, presenting as periventricular echodensities (*arrow in* **a**) that became rapidly progressive over the following days (*arrows in* **b**). She died from severe brain injury with seizures and apneic spells

Timing of CUS	Background

• Serial examinations until discharge
• Routine screening protocol in neonatal units
• Intensify cUS if (suspected) abnormalities
• TEA cUS:
  – GA < 32 weeks
  – Birth weight < 1,500 g
  – Suspected parenchymal brain injury
  – Non-physiological PVE present at discharge
  – IVH grade 3
  – Complications of IVH
  – Meningitis
  – Brain infections
	• Haemorrhagic lesions:
	  – Early detection (hours)
	  – Occur around birth (< 72 h)
	  – Extension first days after event
	  – Later complications (days/weeks)
	• Ischaemic lesions:
	  – Later detection (hours/days after event)
	  – May develop any time during the neonatal period
	  – Early stages may evolve into late, more severe stages over a long period (weeks)
	  – Late detection of end stages
	  – Early stages may seem mild
	  – May be difficult to distinguish from normal phenomena

Appendix 5.1: Ultrasound Screening Protocol

Indications for cUS Examinations

cUS examinations should be performed in:
• Neonates with increased risk of abnormal/delayed brain maturation
• Neonates with increased risk of CNS abnormalities (congenital or acquired)
• Neonates with neurological symptoms

Ultrasound Screening Protocol

I   Preterm (GA ≤32 weeks and/or ≤1,500 g) stable clinical condition and cUS findings

- < 24 h after birth
- Day 3 (including posterior fossa if ≤30 weeks)
- Day 7
- End of the second week
- At postmenstrual age 35 weeks
- Before discharge/transfer
- Around TEA

II   Preterm (GA 32–35 weeks and >1,500 g) stable clinical condition and cUS findings

- Day 3
- Day 7
- At postmenstrual age 35 weeks or before discharge/transfer

III   Preterm (GA <35 weeks) after clinical deterioration (respiratory or circulatory instability, sepsis, necrotizing enterocolitis, apneic spells, etc.)

- < 24 h after the incident
- 3 days after the incident
- 1 week after the incident
- Furthermore: see above

IV   Preterm and P/IVH

- At least every other day in the first week after diagnosis
- In the second week after diagnosis
- Afterwards, if no complications (cerebellar haemorrhage, PHVD, PVHI): see above (I or II)

V   Fullterm and IVH

- At least every other day in the first week after diagnosis
- Afterwards, if no complications: before discharge

VI   IVH and PHVD (regardless of GA)

- Daily until stabilisation PHVD
- Afterwards: weekly until discharge/transfer
- If treatment is necessary: daily until stabilisation

VII   Preterm and non-physiological PVE and/or PVHI

- At least weekly until normalisation
- If cystic lesions develop: weekly until discharge/transfer
- Around TEA

VIII   Hypoxic - ischaemic encephalopathy in (near) term neonate (GA >35 weeks)

- <24 h after birth
- Repeat second day if clinical symptoms and/or cUS abnormalities
- Follow-up until stabilisation or normalisation
- Before discharge/transfer

IX   (suspected) CNS infection

- At onset of clinical symptoms
- Repeat at least every other day until stabilisation without complications

X   Other (admitted to neonatal intensive or high care unit)

- Day 1–3 after admittance
- Repeat if abnormalities seen (see above)

Appendix 5.2: How to Distinguish Physiological from Pathological Echodensities in the White Matter

PVE are likely to be physiological *(see Figs 3.6, 4.3a, 4.5a, b, 5.1a, e and 5.2a)* if:

- The echogenicity is less than the echogenicity of the choroid plexus, and they are:
- Homogeneous

- Symmetric (shape and location)
- Linear
- Well defined
- Of short duration (<7 days) and fading before TEA

PVE are more likely to be non-physiological, indicating white matter injury *(see Figs. 4.5d, e, 5.1b, 5.2b, 5.3a, b)* if:

- The echogenicity is equal to or exceeds that of the choroid plexus.
- The echogenicity extends into the deep white matter *(see Figs 2.4 and 5.5a)* and/or if they are:
- Inhomogeneous
- Asymmetric
- Patchy, less defined
- Of longer duration (≥7 days) and/or persisting beyond TEA

References

Boxma A et al (2005) Sonographic detection of the optic radiation. Acta Paediatr 94(10): 1455–1461

Leijser LM et al (2009a) Frequently encountered cranial ultrasound features in the white matter of preterm infants: correlation with MRI. Eur J Paediatr Neurol 13(4):317–326; Epub 2008 Jul 31

Van Wezel-Meijler G et al (2011a) Diffuse hyperechogenicity of basal ganglia and thalami in preterm neonates: a physiologic finding? Radiology 258:944–50

Van Wezel-Meijler G et al (2011b) Ultrasound detection of white matter injury in very preterm neonates: practical implications. Dev Med Child Neurol 53:29–34

Further Reading

Bracci R et al. (2006) The timing of neonatal brain damage. Biol Neonate 90:145–155

Daneman A et al. (2006) Imaging of the brain in full-term neonates: does sonography still play a role? Pediatr Radiol 36:636–646

De Vries LS et al. (1992) The spectrum of leukomalacia using cranial ultrasound. Behav Brain Res 49:1–6

De Vries LS et al. (2004) Ultrasound abnormalities preceding cerebral palsy in high-risk preterm infants. J Pediatr 144:815–820

De Vries LS et al (2006) The role of cranial ultrasound and magnetic resonance imaging in the diagnosis of infections of the central nervous system. Early Hum Dev 82:819–825; Review

Horsch S et al (2005) Ultrasound diagnosis of brain atrophy is related to neurodevelopmental outcome in preterm infants. Acta Paediatr 94:1815–1821

Leijser LM et al (2008) Comparing brain white matter on sequential cranial ultrasound and MRI in very preterm infants. Neuroradiology 50:799–811

Leijser LM et al (2009b) Brain imaging findings in very preterm infants throughout the neonatal period: Part I. Incidences and evolution of lesions, comparison between ultrasound and MRI. Early Hum Dev 85:101–109

Leijser LM et al (2010) Is sequential cranial ultrasound reliable for detection of white matter injury in very preterm infants? Neuroradiology 52:397–406

Volpe JJ (1989) Intraventricular hemorrhage in the premature infant – current concepts. II. Ann Neurol 25:109–116

Volpe JJ (2008a) Intracranial hemorrhage: subdural, primary subarachnoid, intracerebellar, intraventricular (term infant), and miscellaneous. In: Volpe JJ Neurology of the newborn, 5th edn. Saunders Elsevier, Philadelphia

Volpe JJ (2008b) Intracranial Hemorrhage: Germinal Matrix-Intraventricular Hemorrhage of the Premature Infant. In: Volpe JJ Neurology of the Newborn, 5th edn. Saunders Elsevier, Philadelphia

Scoring Systems

To obtain insight into the severity of lesions and for better prognostication, it is recommended that a scoring system be applied for GMH-IVH, PVE and PVL. These scoring systems are presented in Appendices 6.1–6.3, respectively.

Appendix 6.1: Classification of Germinal Matrix – Intraventricular Haemorrhage

Adapted from Volpe (1989):

- Grade 1: GMH with no or minimal IVH (Fig. 6.1)
- Grade 2: IVH (10–50% of the ventricular area on parasagittal view) (Fig. 6.2, see also Fig. 4.7b)
- Grade 3: IVH (>50% of the ventricular area on parasagittal view, usually distends the lateral ventricle) (Fig. 6.3)
- Separate notation: PHVD (Fig. 6.4, see also Figs. 4.7c and 4.8)
- Separate notation: concomitant periventricular echodensity (including location and extent), referred to as "IPE" (intraparenchymal echodensity), representing PVHI (Fig. 6.5)

G. Meijler, *Neonatal Cranial Ultrasonography*,
DOI 10.1007/978-3-642-21320-5_6,
© Springer-Verlag Berlin Heidelberg 2012

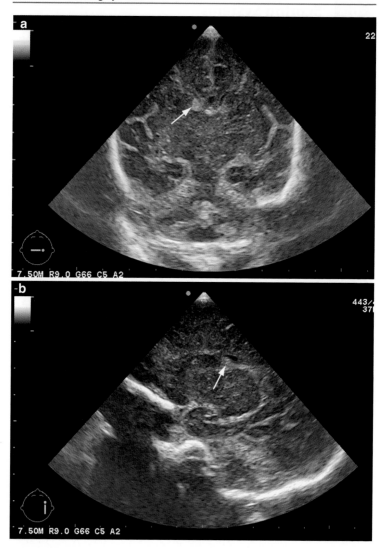

Fig. 6.1 Grade 1 GMH-IVH in a preterm baby (GA 32 weeks, scanned 2 days after birth).
(**a**) Coronal cUS at the level of the frontal horns of the lateral ventricles, showing right-sided GMH (*arrow*; grade 1 GMH-IVH). (**b**) Parasagittal cUS through the right lateral ventricle, also showing the small haemorrhage (*arrow*)

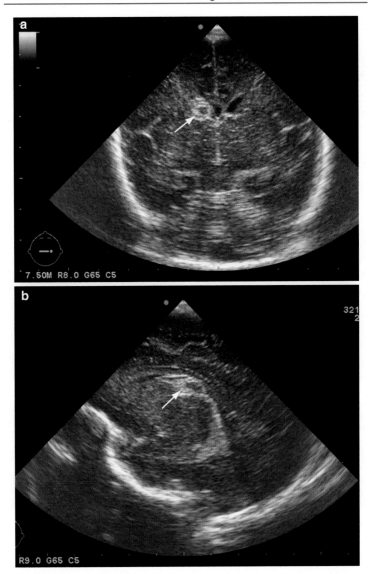

Fig. 6.2 Grade 2 IVH in a very preterm baby (GA 25 + 3 weeks, scanned 3 days after birth). (**a**) Coronal cUS scan, level of the frontal horns of the lateral ventricles, showing right-sided IVH (*arrow*). (**b**) Parasagittal ultrasound scan through right lateral ventricle showing the IVH (*arrow*)

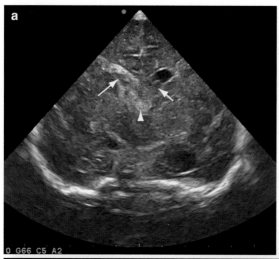

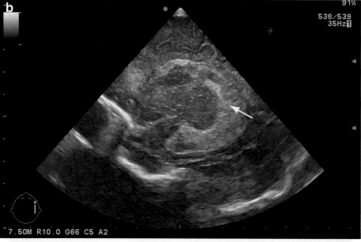

Fig. 6.3 Grade 3 IVH in a near-term neonate born asphyxiated. (**a**) Coronal cUS at the level of the frontal horns of the lateral ventricles, showing large, right-sided IVH (*arrow*) and also small left-sided IVH (*short arrow*) distending the lateral ventricles. Also showing haemorrhage in the 3rd ventricle (*arrowhead*) and echogenic ventricular lining resulting from haemorrhage. (**b**) Parasagittal cUS through the right lateral ventricle, showing the large IVH (*arrow*) which almost completely fills and distends the lateral ventricle

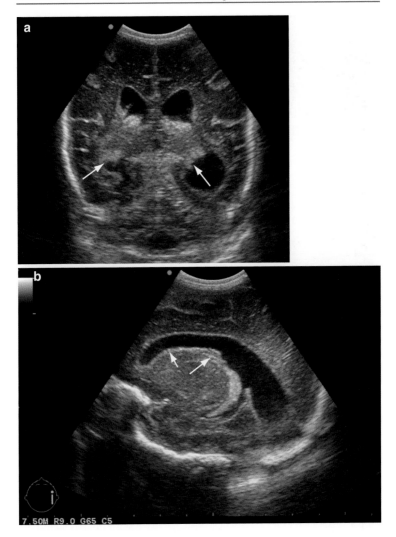

Fig. 6.4 PHVD. Preterm baby, GA 29 + 4 weeks, cUS scan performed at postmenstrual age of 32 weeks. (**a**) Coronal at the level of the trigones of the lateral ventricles, and (**b**) Parasagittal through the lateral ventricle, showing remnants of bilateral IVH (*arrows*), dilatation of the lateral ventricles and echogenic ventricular lining (*short arrow in* **b**)

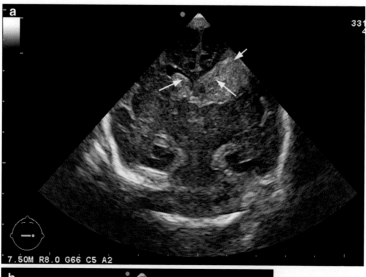

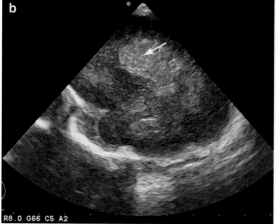

Fig. 6.5 Grade 3 IVH with IPE. Preterm neonate, GA 28 weeks with initially normal cUS scans but large IVH developing 2 days after birth and IPE visible on the third day of life. (**a**) Coronal cUS at the level of the frontal horns of the lateral ventricles, showing bilateral IVH (grade 3) (*arrows*), complicated by a left-sided IPE, representing PVHI (*short arrow*). (**b**) Parasagittal cUS, showing the large IPE in the left fronto-parietal area (*arrow*). (**c**) Coronal cUS at the level of the trigone of the lateral ventricles: after 3 weeks a porencephalic cyst (*arrow*) developed in the area of the IPE. Remnants of the IVH are still visible in the lateral ventricles

Fig. 6.5 (continued)

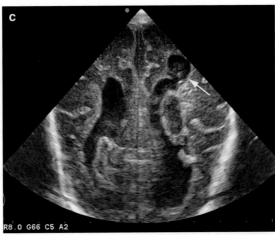

Appendix 6.2: Classification of Periventricular White Matter Echodensity (PVE)

Adapted from van Wezel-Meijler et al. (1998):

- Grade 0 PVE: normal echogenicity of the periventricular white matter (the echogenicity of the periventricular white matter being less than that of the choroid plexus) (Fig. 6.6, see also Figs. 3.3, 3.5, 4.2, 4.6a, b, 4.7a)
- Grade 1 PVE: moderately increased echogenicity of the periventricular white matter, the affected region (or smaller areas within the affected region) being (almost) as bright as the choroid plexus (Figs. 6.7 and 6.8 see also Figs. 3.6, 4.5c, 5.1f)
- Grade 2 PVE: seriously increased echogenicity, the affected region (or smaller areas within the affected region) being brighter than the choroid plexus (Fig. 6.9, also see Figs. 4.5d, e, 5.1b, 5.2b)
- Separate notation: homogeneous, inhomogeneous (For inhomogeneous PVE see Figs. 4.5d, e, 5.1b, f, 5.2b, 5.3a, 6.9)

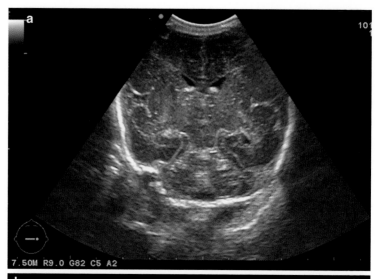

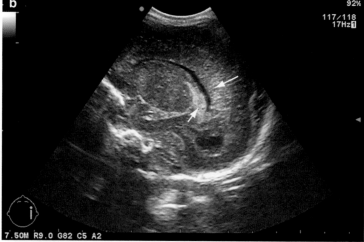

Fig. 6.6 Preterm neonate, GA 28 weeks (same infant as in Fig. 6.5), having normal cUS scan on the first day of life without haemorrhage and with normal echogenicity of the periventricular white matter (*arrow in* **b**), being homogeneous and of lower echogenicity than the choroid plexus (*short arrow in* **b**). (**a**) Coronal scan at the level of the bodies of the lateral ventricles. (**b**) Parasagittal scan through the right lateral ventricle

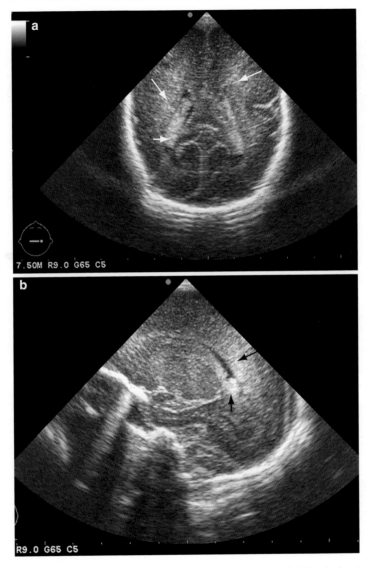

Fig. 6.7 Grade 1 PVE. Preterm neonate, GA 27 + 2 weeks. (**a**) Coronal cUS at the level of the trigone of the lateral ventricles. (**b**) Parasagittal cUS through the left lateral ventricle. The echogenicity of the periventricular white matter (*arrows*) is mildly increased, being almost equal to that of the choroid plexus (*short arrow*)

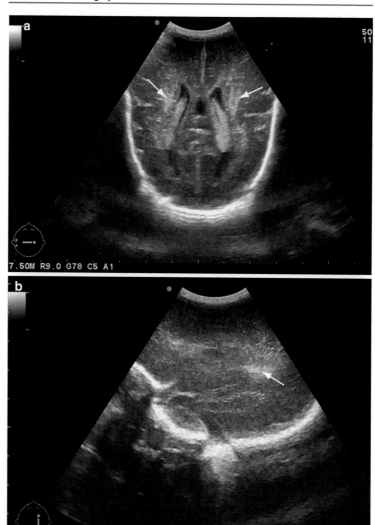

Fig. 6.8 Inhomogeneous grade 1 PVE. Preterm neonate, GA 26 + 2 weeks. (**a**) Coronal cUS at the level of the trigones of the lateral ventricles. (**b**) Parasagittal cUS. The echogenicity of the periventricular white matter is inhomogeneously increased (*arrows*)

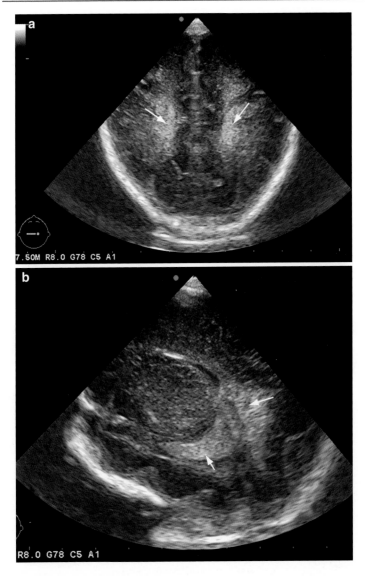

Fig. 6.9 Inhomogeneous grade 2 PVE. Preterm neonate, gestational age 31 + 2 weeks. (**a**) Coronal cUS at the level of the parieto-occipital lobes. (**b**) Parasagittal cUS. The echogenicity of the periventricular white matter is seriously and inhomogeneously increased (*arrows*), exceeding to that of the choroid plexus (*short arrow*). This infant later developed cystic PVL (Fig. 6.11)

Appendix 6.3: Classification of Periventricular Leukomalacia

According to de Vries et al. (1992):

- Grade 1: transient PVE persisting for ≥7 days
- Grade 2: transient PVE evolving into small, localised fronto-parietal cysts (Fig. 6.10)
- Grade 3: PVE evolving into extensive periventricular cystic lesions (Fig. 6.11)
- Grade 4: densities extending into the deep white matter evolving into extensive cystic lesions (Fig. 6.12)

It should be noted that the incidence of "classic" PVL where this classification refers to has importantly declined over the last decade and that there has been a shift towards a more subtle, diffuse form of white matter injury (so-called diffuse white matter injury). For the detection of diffuse white matter injury, MRI is needed as it is not reliably depicted by cUS (see also chapter 5).

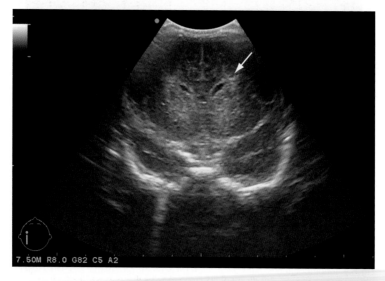

Fig. 6.10 Grade 2 PVL. Preterm neonate, gestational age 27 + 2 weeks. Initially normal cUS scans. cUS performed 4 weeks after birth showing a small, single cystic lesion (*arrow*) in the frontal periventricular white matter on the left side

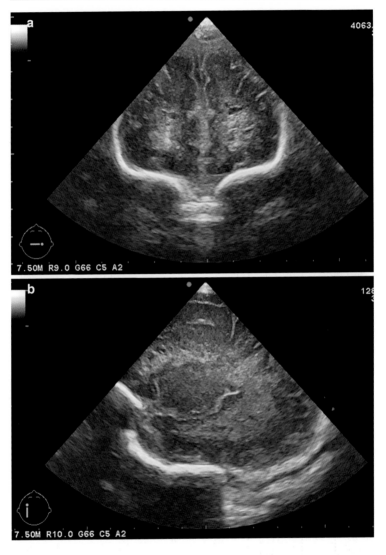

Fig. 6.11 Grade 3 cystic PVL. Preterm neonate, gestational age 31 + 2 weeks, same child as in Fig. 6.9. cUS performed 5 weeks after birth. (**a**) Coronal at the level of the frontal lobes. (**b**) Parasagittal. There are cystic lesions in the fronto-patietal periventricular white matter

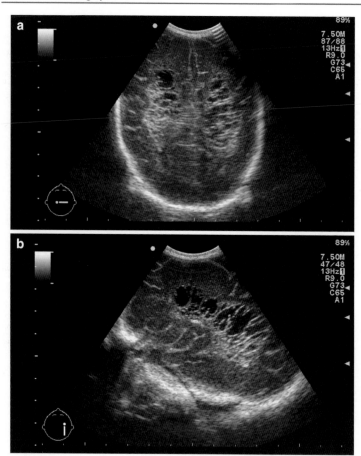

Fig. 6.12 Ultrasound scan in a premature infant who gradually, over a period of weeks, developed extensive leukomalacia (PVL grade 4), showing cystic lesions extending into the deep white matter. This baby was one of monochorionic twins; the pregnancy had been complicated by severe twin-to-twin transfusion syndrome. (**a**) Coronal view at the level of the parieto-occipital lobes. (**b**) Parasagittal view

References

De Vries LS et al (1992) The spectrum of leukomalacia using cranial ultrasound. Behav Brain Res 49:1–6

Van Wezel-Meijler G et al (1998) Magnetic resonance imaging of the brain in premature infants during the neonatal period. Normal phenomena and reflection of mild ultrasound abnormalities. Neuropediatrics 29:89–96

Volpe JJ (1989) Intraventricular hemorrhage in the premature infant – current concepts. II. Ann Neurol 25:109–116

Further Reading

Groenendaal F et al (2010) Complications affecting preterm neonates from 1991 to 2006: what have we gained? Acta Paediatr 99:354–358

Leijser LM et al (2009) Brain imaging findings in very preterm infants throughout the neonatal period: Part I. Incidences and evolution of lesions, comparison between ultrasound and MRI. Early Hum Dev 85:101–109

Leijser LM et al (2010) Is sequential cranial ultrasound reliable for detection of white matter injury in very preterm infants? Neuroradiology 52:397–406

Miller SP et al (2003) Comparing the diagnosis of white matter injury in premature newborns with serial MR imaging and transfontanel ultrasonography findings. AJNR Am J Neuroradiol 24(8):1661–1669

Van Wezel-Meijler G et al (2011) Ultrasound detection of white matter injury in very preterm neonates: practical implications. Dev Med Child Neurol 53 (suppl4):29–34

7.1   Limitations of Cranial Ultrasonography

The advantages of cUS are numerous and widely appreciated (see Chap. 1). It is, however, important to acknowledge the limitations of cUS:

- Image quality can be affected by small acoustic windows, thick hair or hats used for ventilatory support systems. Although the adaptation of transducer frequency to individual situations and the application of additional acoustic windows enhance the possibilities of cUS, some structures and abnormalities remain difficult to visualize.
- The brain's convexity is not well visualized: (small) arterial cortical infarctions and watershed lesions may be overlooked, especially in the first days after the event; subtle aspects of cortical folding will not be reliably assessed, and extracerebral haemorrhage located at the convexity of the cerebral hemispheres (i.e. subdural, epidural, and subarachnoid haemorrhages) may remain beyond the scope of cUS.
- Hypoglycaemic parenchymal injury, often involving the occipital lobes, may not be recognized unless cUS is performed through the posterior fontanel.
- Some lesions resulting from infection, such as (micro-) abscesses and encephalitis, may not be optimally recognized by cUS.
- Cerebellar haemorrhage and other acquired or congenital abnormalities of the cerebellum may have important consequences for neurodevelopment. These and other posterior fossa abnormalities are usually detected, especially if additional scanning is performed through the posterior and/or mastoid fontanels. It is, however, not always possible to define abnormalities precisely and to determine the exact location and extent of abnormalities.

G. Meijler, *Neonatal Cranial Ultrasonography*,
DOI 10.1007/978-3-642-21320-5_7,
© Springer-Verlag Berlin Heidelberg 2012

- Myelination is not visualised. Involvement of the (posterior limb of the) internal capsule in lesions, of major importance for neurological outcome, cannot be determined with certainty by cUS.
- Injury to the basal ganglia in term hypoxic-ischaemic encephalopathy and areas of focal infarction are usually detected, but they may not be defined well enough for accurate prognostication.
- Diffuse white matter injury, frequently occurring in very preterm infants, is not reliably detected by CUS.

7.2   Role of MRI

Although MRI cannot replace serial cUS, there are many conditions requiring MRI. MRI depicts brain maturation, including myelination, in detail. MRI helps to define pathological processes and enables prognostication in many cases. It helps to establish the precise site, origin and extent of lesions. If abnormalities exist in areas that are difficult to access with cUS, MRI may detect lesions that cUS does not. MRI allows detection of diffuse and non-cystic white matter lesions in preterm infants. Modern MRI techniques allow very early detection of hypoxic-ischaemic brain injury and of flow in the cerebral vessels. Measurements of diffusivity enable quantification of maturation and injury, while volume measurements enable quantification of brain growth and tissue loss. However, MRI does not allow for frequent, serial imaging, and very early imaging within a few hours after birth is hard to realize. In addition, although safe, MRI is more burdening than cUS for the sick and/or preterm neonate. Some conditions, such as calcifications, germinolytic cysts and lenticulostriate vasculopathy, are better or only depicted by ultrasound.

Thus, in modern neonatology, cUS and MRI are used as complementary neuroimaging tools.

7.2.1   Conditions in Which MRI Contributes to Diagnosis and/or Prognosis

- Term hypoxic-ischaemic encephalopathy
- Prematurity, gestational age <30 weeks (reliable detection of white matter and cerebellar injury)

- Full-term infant presenting with seizures
- Other neurological symptoms, insufficiently explained by cUS findings
- Arterial infarction (exact location and extent)
- Supratentorial parenchymal abnormalities as seen by cUS
- Infratentorial abnormalities as seen by cUS
- Congenital or acquired infections of the central nervous system
- Congenital malformations of the central nervous system
- Subdural or subarachnoid haemorrhage
- Hypoglycaemia in the presence of seizures
- Metabolic disease
- Severe posthaemorrhagic ventricular dilatation (for reliable assessment of the white matter)
- Periventricular haemorrhagic infarction (exact location and extent)
- Sinovenous Thrombosis
- (Suspected) Abnormalities at the brain's convexity

In Appendix 7.1, indications for MRI are presented.

7.3   Role of CT

The radiation dose involved in CT scanning is significant and in most cases CT has little or no additional diagnostic value when utilized for brain imaging, when compared to high quality cUS and MRI. Therefore, neonatal cerebral CT should only be applied for rare conditions. These include suspected calcifications at the brain's convexity, acute subdural or subarachnoid haemorrhages if intervention is considered and MRI is not readily available and skull fractures following significant traumatic birth. CT Venography may be necessary if cUS or MR Venography are non-diagnostic and there is a need to include or exclude a sinovenous thrombosis.

Appendix 7.1: Indications for Neonatal MRI Examinations

- Preterm birth, GA <30 weeks (preferably around TEA), except in cases without cUS abnormalities (van Wezel-Meijler et al. 2011);

- GMH-IVH > grade 2 (preferably around TEA) (Volpe 1989);
- Hypoxic-ischaemic encephalopathy in (near) term neonates (GA ≥ 35 weeks) (preferably 4–5 days after the incident);
- (cUS) suspicion of Parenchymal brain injury;
- (cUS) suspicion of Posterior fossa abnormalities;
- (cUS) suspicion of Sinovenous thrombosis;
- (cUS suspicion of) extracerebral haemorrhage;
- Symptomatic and/or long lasting and/or recurrent hypoglycaemia;
- Seizures;
- CNS infection with neurological symptoms and/or cUS abnormalities;
- Metabolic disorder with neurological symptoms and/or cUS abnormalities;
- (cUS) Suspicion of Kernicterus;
- (cUS) Suspicion of congenital CNS anomalies

References

Van Wezel-Meijler G et al (2011) Ultrasound detection of white matter injury in very preterm neonates: practical implications Dev Med Child Neurol 53 (suppl4): 29–34

Volpe JJ (1989) Intraventricular hemorrhage in the premature infant – current concepts. II. Ann Neurol 25:109–116

Further Reading

Berfelo FJ, et al (2008) Neonatal cerebral sinovenous thrombosis from symptom to outcome. Stroke 41(7):1382–1388

Burns CM et al (2008) Patterns of cerebral injury and neurodevelopmental outcomes after symptomatic neonatal hypoglycemia. Pediatrics 122:65–74

Cowan F et al (2005) Does cranial ultrasound imaging identify arterial cerebral infarction in term neonates? Arch Dis Child Fetal Neonatal Ed 90:F252–F256

Daneman A et al (2006) Imaging of the brain in full-term neonates: does sonography still play a role? Pediatr Radiol 36:636–646

De Vries LS et al (1999) Asymmetrical myelination of the posterior limb of the internal capsule in infants with periventricular haemorrhagic infarction: an early predictor of hemiplegia. Neuropediatrics 30:314–319

De Vries LS et al (2006) The role of cranial ultrasound and magnetic resonance imaging in the diagnosis of infections of the central nervous system. Early Hum Dev 82:819–825

De Vries LS, Cowan FM (2007) Should cranial MRI screening of preterm infants become routine? Nat Rev Neurol 3:532–533

De Vries LS et al (2011) Myth: cerebral palsy cannot be predicted by neonatal brain imaging. Semin Fetal Neonatal Med 16:279–287

Kersbergen KJ et al (2011) The spectrum of associated brain lesions in cerebral sinovenous thrombosis: relation to gestational age and outcome. Arch Dis Child Fetal Neonatal Ed. 11:96(6):F404–F409

Leijser LM et al (2009) Brain imaging findings in very preterm infants throughout the neonatal period: part I. Incidences and evolution of lesions, comparison between ultrasound and MRI. Early Hum Dev 85:101–109

Leijser LM et al (2010) Is sequential cranial ultrasound reliable for detection of white matter injury in very preterm infants? Neuroradiology 52:397–406

Limperopoulos C et al (2005) Cerebellar hemorrhage in the preterm infant: ultrasonographic findings and risk factors. Pediatrics 116:717–724

Limperopoulos C et al (2009) Cerebellar injury in term infants: clinical characteristics, magnetic resonance imaging findings, and outcome. Pediatr Neurol 41:1–8

Mathur AM, Neil JJ, Inder TE (2010) Understanding brain injury and neurodevelopmental disabilities in the preterm infant: the evolving role of advanced magnetic resonance imaging. Semin Perinatol 34:57–66

Miller SP, Ferriero DM (2009) From selective vulnerability to connectivity: insights from newborn brain imaging. Trends Neurosci 32:496–505

Ramenghi LA et al (2009) Neonatal cerebral sinovenous thrombosis. Semin Fetal Neonatal Med 14:278–283

Rutherford MA et al (1998) Abnormal magnetic resonance signal in the internal capsule predicts poor neurodevelopmental outcome in infants with hypoxic-ischemic encephalopathy. Pediatrics 102:323–328

Rutherford M (ed) (2002) MRI of the neonatal brain. WB Saunders, London

Rutherford MA et al (2005) Advanced MR techniques in the term-born neonate with perinatal brain injury. Semin Fetal Neonatal Med 10:445–460

Steggerda SJ et al (2009a) Cerebellar injury in preterm infants: incidence and findings on US and MR images. Radiology 252(1):190–199

Steggerda SJ, Leijser L, Walther FJ, van Wezel-Meijler G (2009b) Neonatal Cranial Ultrasonography: how to optimize its performance. Early Hum Dev 85:93–99

Van Wezel-Meijler G et al (2009) Magnetic resonance imaging of the brain in newborn infants: practical aspects. Early Hum Dev 85(2):85–92

8.1   Maturational Processes

During the late foetal and the perinatal period and during early infancy, major maturational processes and growth of the brain take place (Volpe 2008). Because of this ongoing maturation, the preterm brain in particular is very vulnerable to deviant development and injury. Patterns of perinatal brain injury depend not only on the origin of the injury (i.e. traumatic, hypoxic-ischaemic, inflammatory, haemorrhagic, etc.) but also on the age of the foetus or infant at the time of the event(s) (Miller et al. 2005; Miller and Ferriero 2009).

Maturational phenomena give specific cUS features, and cUS images change with ongoing maturation (see Chap. 5). Those performing neonatal cUS need to be well informed about normal brain maturation, maturational phenomena as depicted with cUS, and age-related patterns of perinatal brain injury.

Some of the maturational processes can be visualized by modern cUS techniques, resulting in age-specific features, and will be reviewed in this chapter.

8.2   Gyration

Gyration starts in the second trimester of pregnancy; continues in an ordered, predictable way; and is completed around term age when the brain surface has an almost mature appearance. In extremely preterm infants (GA

G. Meijler, *Neonatal Cranial Ultrasonography*,
DOI 10.1007/978-3-642-21320-5_8,
© Springer-Verlag Berlin Heidelberg 2012

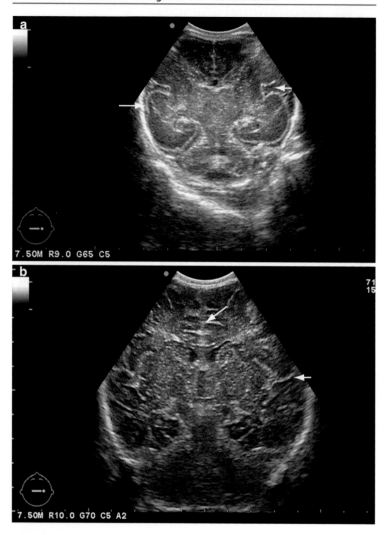

Fig. 8.1 (**a** and **b**) cUS scan at the level of the frontal horns of the lateral ventricles. (**a**) Very preterm neonate (GA 26 weeks), showing very smooth cortex (*arrow*) and open insulae (*short arrow*); (**b**) term infant showing advanced cortical folding (*arrow*) and closed insulae (*short arrow*)

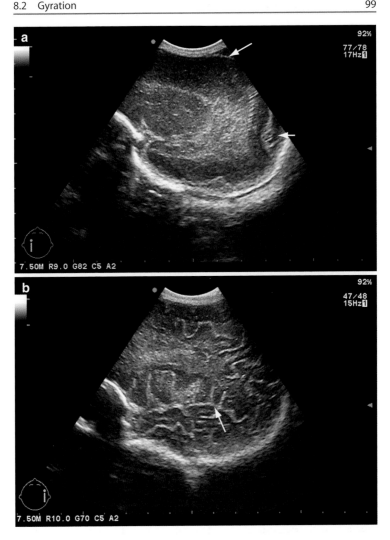

Fig. 8.2 (**a** and **b**) Parasagittal cUS scan at the level of the insula. (**a**) Very preterm infant, showing a smooth cortex (*arrow*) and absent gyration of the insular cortex. Also shows wide subarachnoid space (*short arrow*). (**b**) Full-term infant, showing advanced development of the insular cortex (*arrow*)

24–26 weeks), the brain surface is still very smooth and has a lissencephalic appearance (Figs. 8.1 and 8.2) (van der Knaap et al. 1996).

There are striking regional differences in gyral development: The posterior regions of the brain develop much faster than the anterior regions. Thus, at around 34 weeks of gestation, the frontal cortex is still very smooth, while the occipital cortex already shows obvious gyration. The process of gyration can be followed by cUS. It is possible to assess the GA of the infant from the ultrasound images.

cUS images of very preterm infants before term age differ substantially from those obtained in infants of around term age, mainly because of the difference in gyration (see Figs. 8.1 and 8.2).

While obvious differences in cortical folding as seen on cUS between preterm and full-term infants have not been reported, MRI studies have shown that cortical development is not as complex around TEA in infants born very prematurely as it is in full-term controls.

8.3   Cell Migration

In the first trimester of pregnancy neurons migrate towards the immature cortex. Although neuronal cell migration is completed after 20 weeks of gestation, migration of glial cells continues until late gestation.

In normal preterm infants, subtle areas of symmetrically increased echogenicity, mainly in the frontal regions, can be recognised on cUS images. These areas of increased echogenicity (Fig. 8.3) represent glial cell migration and should be distinguished from non-physiological frontal PVE (van Wezel-Meijler et al. 1998) (see Figs. 5.1a and b, 5.3 and Chap. 5).

8.4   Germinal Matrix Involution

The germinal matrix is an abundant, highly cellular and vascular "strip" of subependymal tissue. During early gestation, it lines the entire wall of the lateral ventricles and third ventricle. It produces neuroblasts and glioblasts and is the origin of migrating neurons (first trimester) and glial cells

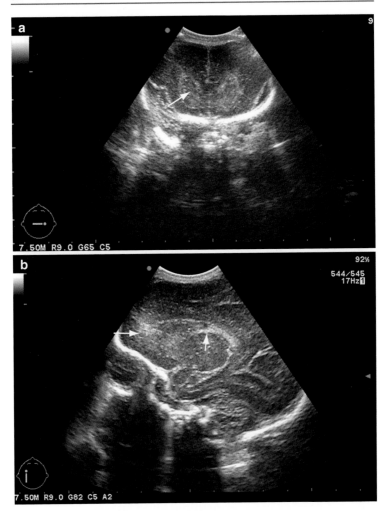

Fig. 8.3 (**a**) Coronal cUS scan at the level of the frontal horns and (**b**) parasagittal cUS scan in very preterm infant (GA 26 weeks), showing symmetric, homogeneously increased echogenicity in the frontal white matter (*arrows*), being a normal finding in preterm neonates before TEA. *Short arrow* in (**b**) indicates remnants of the germinal matrix

(second and third trimesters). Regression of the germinal matrix starts from 24 to 26 weeks gestation onwards. After 34 weeks, remnants remain in the thalamo-caudate notch and temporal horns of the lateral ventricles. On cUS, the germinal matrix can be distinguished as small areas of high echogenicity, mostly only visible on parasagittal scans, around the thalamo-caudate notch (see Fig. 8.3) (van Wezel-Meijler et al. 1998). These small echogenic areas should be distinguished from GMH (see Fig. 6.1b).

8.5   Deep Grey Matter Changes

Serial cUS in preterm infants shows changes over time in the thalami and basal ganglia. In very preterm infants, these deep grey matter structures may show diffuse, subtly increased echogenicity as compared to the surrounding tissue (Fig. 8.4). It is generally more outspoken in the basal ganglia than the thalami, is seen in about 90% of very preterm infants (GA < 32 weeks), fades with age and is generally no longer seen after 1 month post-term (van Wezel-Meijler et al. 2011).

This normal prematurity-related cUS phenomenon should be distinguished from pathological changes in the deep grey matter, typically occurring in (near)-term neonates after perinatal asphyxia. These changes may also be subtle and diffuse, but represent hypoxic-ischaemic injury and may be of great clinical importance (Fig. 8.5 see also Figs. 2.2b, 2.3 and 4.6c, d). It should also be distinguished from more localised or unilateral lesions in the thalami and/or basal ganglia, resulting from haemorrhage or infarction in these areas (see Fig. 4.6e).

8.6   Changes in Cerebrospinal Fluid Spaces

In the foetus and very preterm infant, the lateral ventricles are often wide and asymmetric (usually the left is larger than the right) with very wide occipital horns (Fig. 8.6). Subarachnoid spaces may also be wide (Fig. 8.7; see also Fig. 8.2a). Because of brain growth and fluid loss in the first few days after birth, the cerebrospinal fluid spaces gradually become smaller.

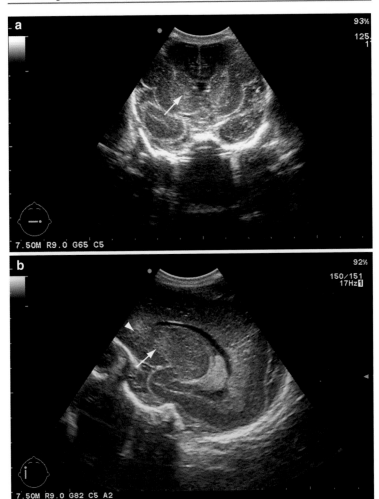

Fig. 8.4 (**a**) Coronal cUS scan at the level of the frontal horns of the lateral ventricles and (**b**) parasagittal cUS scan in very preterm infant (same infant as Fig. 8.3), showing subtle, diffuse echogenicity of the basal ganglia (*arrows*) being a normal finding in preterm neonates before TEA. Also showing physiological frontal echodensity (*arrowhead*)

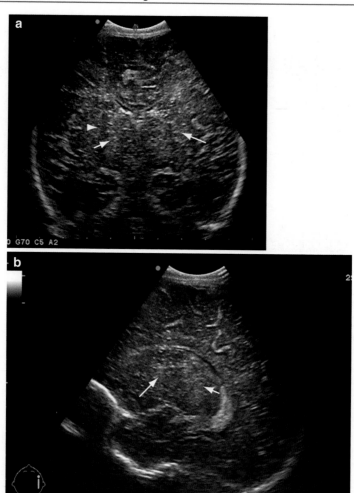

Fig. 8.5 (**a**) Coronal cUS scan at the level of the bodies of the lateral ventricles and (**b**) parasagittal cUS scan in full-term neonate born asphyxiated (scanning performed on the 2nd day of life), showing subtle increased echogenicity in the area of the basal ganglia (*arrow*) and thalami (*short arrow*), representing hypoxic-ischemic injury at this age. On the coronal image, the internal capsule can be recognized as low echogenicity structure between the basal ganglia and thalamus (*arrowhead*). This phenomenon can be recognized in neonates with hypoxic-ischaemic injury of the deep gray matter

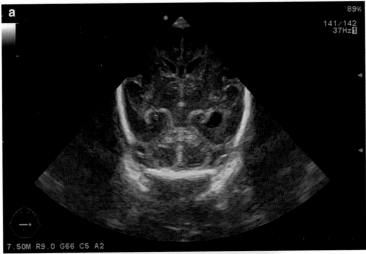

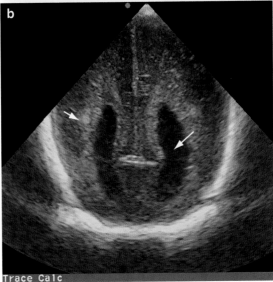

Fig. 8.6 (**a** and **b**) Coronal and (**c**) parasagittal cUS scan in very preterm neonate (GA 25 weeks) at respectively the level of the frontal horns of the lateral ventricles, the parieto-occipital lobes and through the left lateral ventricle, showing wide and asymmetric lateral ventricles and the very prominent occipital horns (normal at this age) (*arrows*). Also showing in (**b**) abnormally increased echogenicity (*PVE*) in the right parietal area (*short arrow*)

Fig. 8.6 (continued)

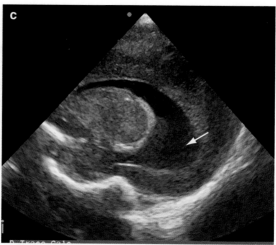

Under some conditions (after extreme prematurity, in infants with congenital cardiac defects, and hypoxic-ischaemic brain injury the cerebrospinal fluid spaces remain or become wide, even after term age (Fig. 8.8 see also Fig. 4.9). This may be the result of impaired brain growth.

Changes of brain maturation
• Increase in volume and weight
• Cortical folding
• Myelination
• Cell migration
• Germinal matrix involution
• Deep grey matter changes
• Decrease in cerebrospinal fluid spaces

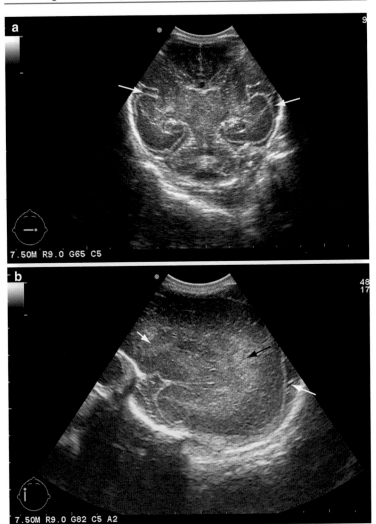

Fig. 8.7 (a) Coronal cUS scan at the level of the bodies of the lateral ventricles and (b) parasagittal CUS scan through the insula in very preterm neonate (same infant as Figs. 8.3 and 8.4), showing wide subarachnoid spaces (*arrows*), also showing the open Sylvian fissures (*short arrow in* **a**), frontal echodensity (*short arrow in* **b**) (normal phenomena at this age) and grade 1 PVE in (**b**) (*black arrow*)

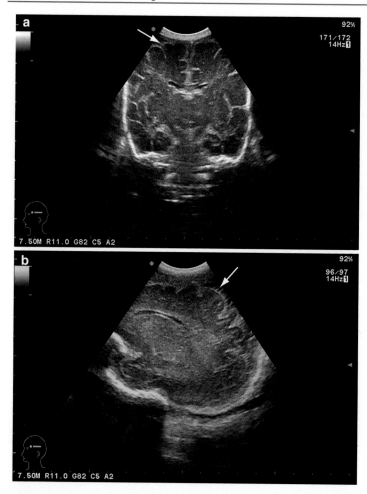

Fig. 8.8 (a) Coronal cUS scan at the level of the bodies of the lateral ventricles and (b) parasagittal cUS scan in very preterm neonate (GA 27 + 6 weeks, scanned around TEA), showing wide subarachnoid spaces (*arrows*), probably resulting from impaired brain growth

References

Miller SP et al (2005) Patterns of brain injury in term neonatal encephalopathy. J Pediatr 146(4):453–60

Miller SP, Ferriero DM. (2009) From selective vulnerability to connectivity: insights from newborn brain imaging. Trends Neurosci 32(9):496–505. Epub 2009 Aug 25

Van der Knaap MS et al (1996) Normal gyration and sulcation in preterm and term neonates: appearance on MR images. Radiology 200:389–396

Van Wezel-Meijler G et al (1998) Magnetic resonance imaging of the brain in premature infants during the neonatal period. Normal phenomena and reflection of mild ultrasound abnormalities. Neuropediatrics 29:89–96

Van Wezel-Meijler G et al (2011) Diffuse hyperechogenicity of the basal ganglia and thalami in preterm infants: a physiological finding? Radiology 258(3):944–950

Volpe JJ (2008) Neuronal proliferation, migration, organization and myelination. In: Neurology of the newborn. WB Saunders, Philadelphia; Bildlegenden

Further Reading

Brouwer MJ et al (2010) Ultrasound measurements of the lateral ventricles in neonates: why, how and when? A systematic review. Acta Paediatr 99(9):1298–1306

Brouwer MJ et al (2012) New reference values for the neonatal cerebral ventricles. Radiology 262(1):224–233. Epub 2011

Chi JG et al (1977) Gyral development of the human brain. Ann Neurol 1:86–93

Childs AM, Ramenghi LA, Cornette L et al (2001) Cerebral maturation in premature infants: quantitative assessment using MR imaging. AJNR Am J Neuroradiol 22:1577–1582

Cowan F (2002) Magnetic resonance imaging of the normal infant brain: term to 2 years. In: Rutherford M (ed) MRI of the neonatal brain. WB Saunders, London

Huppi PS et al (1996) Structural and neurobehavioral delay in postnatal brain development of preterm infants. Pediatr Res 39:895–901

Larroche J-C (1987) Le developpement du cerveau foetal humain. Atlas anatomique. INSERM, CNRS, Paris

Leijser LM et al (2009) Frequently encountered cranial ultrasound features in the white matter of preterm infants: correlation with MRI. Eur J Paediatr Neurol 13(4): 317–326

Murphy NP et al (1989) Cranial ultrasound assessment of gestational age in low birthweight infants. Arch Dis Child 64:569–572

Naidich TP et al (1994) The developing cerebral surface. Preliminary report on the patterns of sulcal and gyral maturation – anatomy, ultrasound, and magnetic resonance imaging. Neuroimaging Clin N Am 4:201–240

Veyrac C et al (2006) Brain ultrasonography in the premature infant. Pediatr Radiol 36:626–635

- cUS is an essential diagnostic tool in modern neonatology. It is very suitable for screening, and it depicts normal anatomy and maturational and pathological changes in the brains of preterm and full-term neonates. cUS can only reliably be performed by specially trained individuals using suitable equipment and techniques. cUS plays an important role in predicting neurological prognosis in the high-risk newborn.
- Standard cUS is performed using the anterior fontanel as acoustic window. The whole brain is scanned, and images are recorded in at least six coronal and five sagittal planes with a scan frequency of 7.5-MHz. In individual cases other scan frequencies may need to be applied, and scanning through supplemental acoustic windows may be necessary.
- Optimal timing and frequency of serial cUS examinations is essential. It is recommended that screening protocols be applied in neonatal units. Screening schedules should take into account that in the high-risk neonate ischaemic lesions may develop at any time during the neonatal period and may change in appearance over a variable period of time.
- MRI is recommended in the case of (suspected) parenchymal brain injury and in very preterm neonates, neonates with neurological symptoms, congenital malformations and miscellaneous disorders. MRI helps to define pathological processes, can show the location and extent of lesions more precisely, better depicts abnormalities in the posterior fossa, shows preterm white matter injury and enables prognostication in many cases. In addition, MRI gives more detailed information about maturational processes.

G. Meijler, *Neonatal Cranial Ultrasonography,*
DOI 10.1007/978-3-642-21320-5_9,
© Springer-Verlag Berlin Heidelberg 2012

- Knowledge of normal brain anatomy and maturation is essential when performing cUS, and maturational changes need to be distinguished from (mild) pathology.
- Patterns of perinatal brain injury depend, among others, on the origin of the injury and on the postmenstrual age of the infant.

PART II

ULTRASOUND ANATOMY OF THE NEONATAL BRAIN

The ultrasound scans shown in this section are normal, considering the GA of the infant and the post menstrual age (PMA) at scanning, unless stated otherwise.

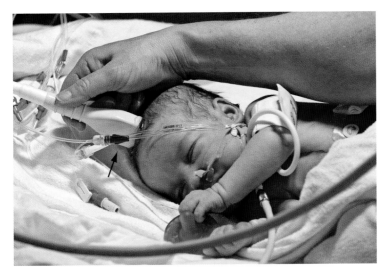

Fig. 10.1 Probe positioning for obtaining coronal planes (*arrow* indicates marker on transducer)

Fig. 10.2 Coronal plane

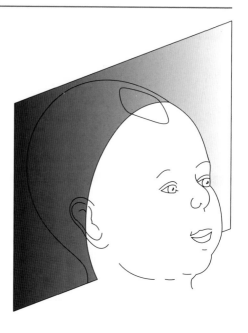

Fig. 10.3 Standard six coronal planes

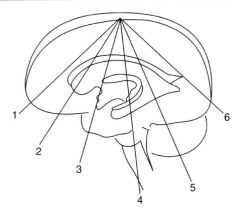

Legends of Corresponding Numbers in Ultrasound Scans (C1)

1. Interhemispheric fissure
2. Frontal lobe
3. Skull
4. Orbit

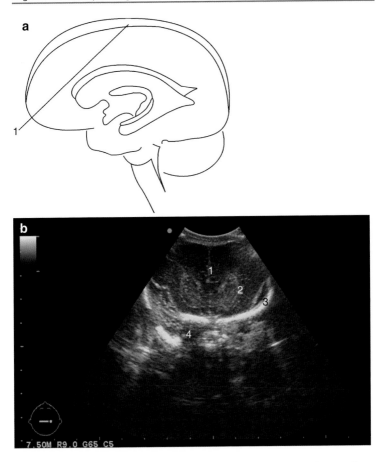

Fig. 10.4 (**a**) First coronal plane (C1) at the level of the frontal lobes. (**b**) Ultrasound scan of the first coronal plane (C1) at the level of the frontal lobes (GA and PMA 26 + 2 weeks). Image shows symmetric echogenicity of the frontal white matter (frontal echodensities), a normal finding in preterm neonates before TEA (see Part I, Chap. 8)

Legends of Corresponding Numbers in Ultrasound Scans (C2)

1. Interhemispheric fissure
2. Frontal Lobe
5. Frontal horn of lateral ventricle
6. Caudate Nucleus
7. Basal ganglia
8. Temporal Lobe
9. Sylvian fissure
10. Corpus callosum
11. Cavum septum pellucidum

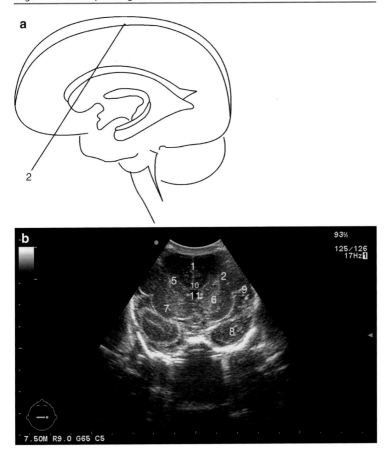

Fig. 10.5 (**a**) Second coronal plane (C2) at the level of the frontal horns of the lateral ventricles. (**b**) Ultrasound scan of the second coronal plane (C2) at the level of the frontal horns of the lateral ventricles (same infant as Fig. 1.4b). Image shows narrow lateral ventricles, a normal finding in a normal appearing brain. Also showing subtle, symmetric echogenicity of the caudate nuclei, a normal finding in preterm neonates before TEA (see Part I, Chap. 8)

Legends of Corresponding Numbers in Ultrasound Scans (C3)

1. Interhemispheric fissure
2. Frontal lobe
3. Skull
5. Frontal horn of lateral ventricle
6. Caudate nucleus
7. Basal ganglia
8. Temporal lobe
9. Sylvian fissure
10. Corpus callosum
11. Cavum septum pellucidum
12. Third ventricle
13. Cingulate gyrus

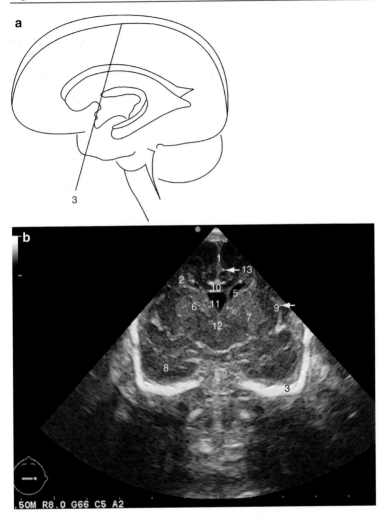

Fig. 10.6 (**a**) Third coronal plane (C3) at the level of foramen of Monroe and the 3rd ventricle. (**b**) Ultrasound scan of the third coronal plane (C3) at the level of foramen of Monroe and the 3rd ventricle (GA 25 + 4 weeks, PMA 26 +3 weeks)

Legends of Corresponding Numbers in Ultrasound Scans (C4)

1. Interhemispheric fissure
2. Frontal lobe
3. Skull
6. Caudate nucleus
7. Basal ganglia
8. Temporal lobe
9. Sylvian fissure
11. Cavum septum pellucidum
12. Third ventricle
14. Body lateral ventricle

15. Choroid plexus
    (*: plexus in third ventricle)
16. Thalamus
17. Hippocampal fissure
18. Mesencephalic aqueduct
19a. Cerebellar hemisphere
19b. Cerebellar vermis
20. Temporal horn of lateral ventricle
21. Tentorium
22. Parietal lobe

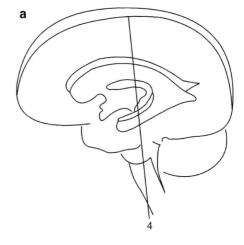

Fig. 10.7 (**a**) Fourth coronal plane (C4) at the level of the body of the lateral ventricles. (**b**) Ultrasound scan of the fourth coronal plane (C4) at the level of the body of the lateral ventricles (GA 25 + 5 weeks, PMA 26 + 5 weeks). (**b′**) Ultrasound scan of the fourth coronal plane (C4), at the level of the body of the lateral ventricles slightly more occipital than in Fig. 1.7b (GA and PMA 26 +2 weeks)

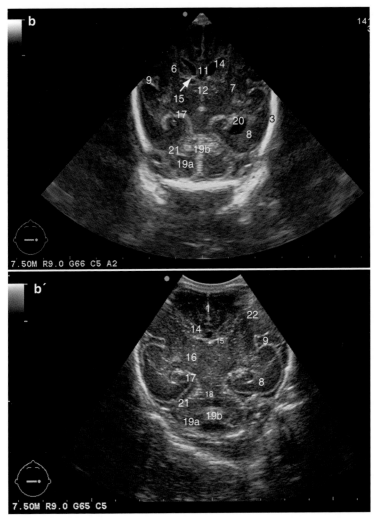

Fig. 10.7 (continued)

Legends of Corresponding Numbers in Ultrasound Scans (C5)

1. Interhemispheric fissure
3. Skull
8. Temporal lobe
9. Sylvian fissure
10. Corpus callosum
15. Choroid plexus
22. Parietal lobe
23. Occipital horn of lateral ventricle

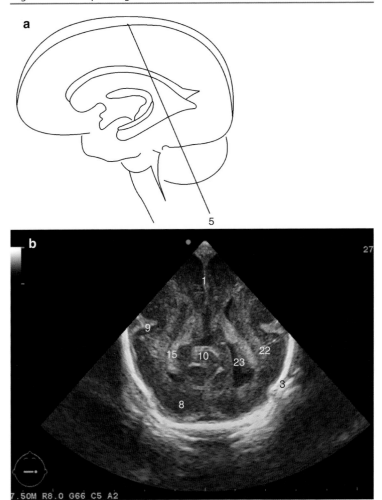

Fig. 10.8 (**a**) Fifth coronal plane (C5) at the level of the trigone of the lateral ventricles. (**b**) Ultrasound scan of the fifth coronal plane (C5) at the level of the trigone of the lateral ventricles (GA 25 + 4 weeks, PMA 25 + 6 weeks)

Legends of Corresponding Numbers in Ultrasound Scans (C6)

1. Interhemispheric fissure
9. Sylvian fissure
22. Parietal lobe
24. Parieto-occipital fissure
25. Occipital lobe

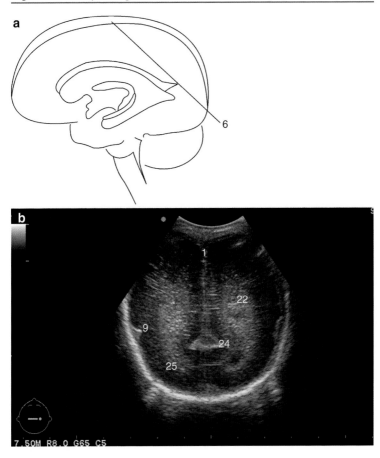

Fig. 10.9 (**a**) Sixth coronal plane (C6) through the occipital lobes. (**b**) Ultrasound scan of the sixth coronal plane (C6) at the level of the occipital lobes (GA and PMA 27 + 2 weeks). Image shows mild, homogeneous echogenicity of the parietal white matter: PVE grade 1 (homogeneous) (see Part I, Chap. 6)

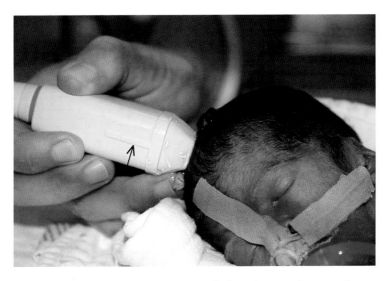

Fig. 11.1 Probe positioning to obtain sagittal planes (*arrow* indicates marker on transducer)

Fig. 11.2 Sagittal plane

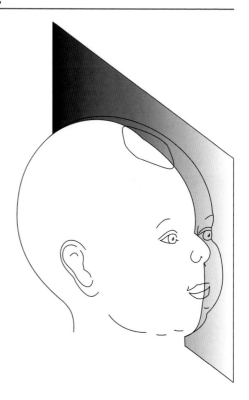

Fig. 11.3 Standard five sagittal
planes

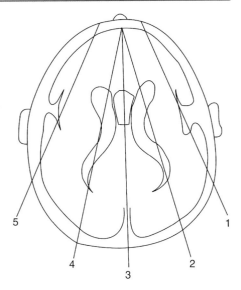

Legends of Corresponding Numbers in Ultrasound Scans (S3)

10. Corpus callosum
11. Cavum septum pellucidum
12. Third ventricle
13. Cingulate gyrus
19b. Cerebellar vermis
26. Calcarine fissure
28. Pons

29. Medulla oblongata
30. → Fourth ventricle
31. Cisterna magna
32. Cisterna quadrigemina
33. Interpeduncular fossa
34. Fornix

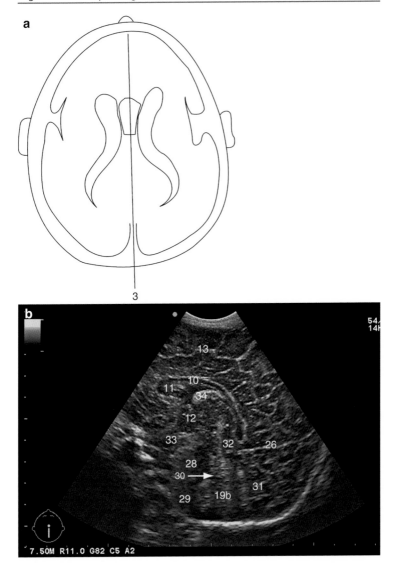

Fig. 11.4 (a) Midsagittal plane (S3) through corpus callosum, 3rd and 4th ventricle. (b) Ultrasound scan of midsagittal plane (S3) through 3rd and 4th ventricle (full-term neonate)

Legends of Corresponding Numbers in Ultrasound Scans (S2, S4)

2. Frontal lobe
5. Frontal horn of lateral ventricle
6. Caudate nucleus
8. Temporal lobe
14. Body lateral ventricle
15. Choroid plexus
16. Thalamus
17. Hippocampal fissure

19a. Cerebellar hemisphere
20. Temporal horn of lateral ventricle
22. Parietal lobe
23. Trigone of lateral ventricle
25. Occipital lobe
35. Occipital horn of lateral ventricle

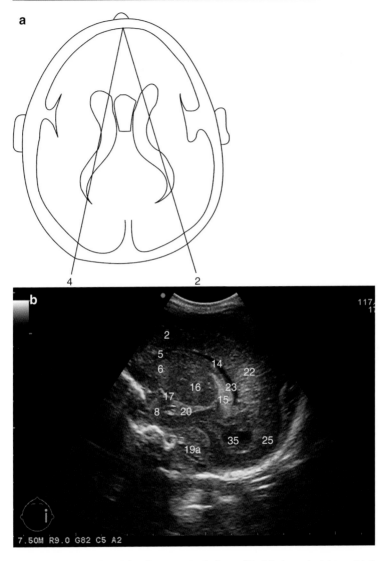

Fig. 11.5 (**a**) Second and fourth parasagittal planes (S2, S4) through right and left lateral ventricles. (**b**) Ultrasound scan of fourth parasagittal planes (S4) through right lateral ventricle (GA 27 + 3 weeks, PMA 27 + 3 weeks)

Legends of Corresponding Numbers in Ultrasound Scans (S1, S5)

2. Frontal lobe
8. Temporal lobe
9. Sylvian fissure

22. Parietal lobe
25. Occipital lobe
36. Insula

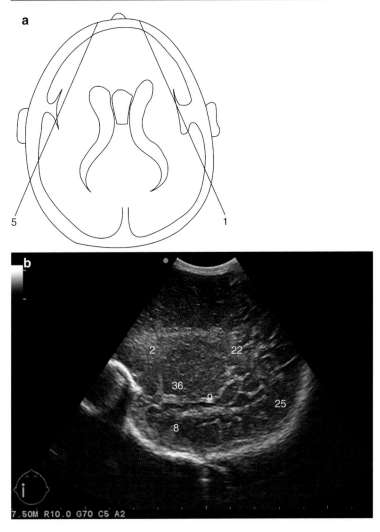

Fig. 11.6 (**a**) First and fifth parasagittal plane (S1, S5) through insulae (*right* and *left*). (**b**) Ultrasound scan of fifth parasagittal planes (S5) through left insula (full-term neonate)

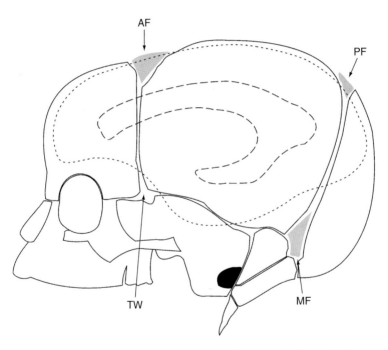

Fig. 12.1 The acoustic windows. *AF* anterior fontanel, *PF* posterior fontanel, *TW* temporal window, *MF* mastoid (or posterolateral) fontanel

G. Meijler, *Neonatal Cranial Ultrasonography,*
DOI 10.1007/978-3-642-21320-5_12,
© Springer-Verlag Berlin Heidelberg 2012

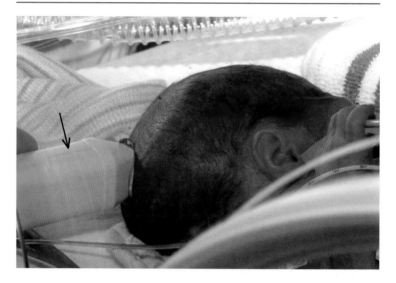

Fig. 12.2 Probe position to obtain coronal view, using the posterior fontanel as the acoustic window (*arrow* indicates marker)

Legends of Corresponding Numbers in Ultrasound Scans

8. Temporal lobe

19a. Cerebellar hemisphere

19b. Cerebellar vermis

21. Tentorium

25. Occipital lobe

29. Medulla oblongata

30. Fourth ventricle

35. Occipital horn of lateral ventricle

37. Falx

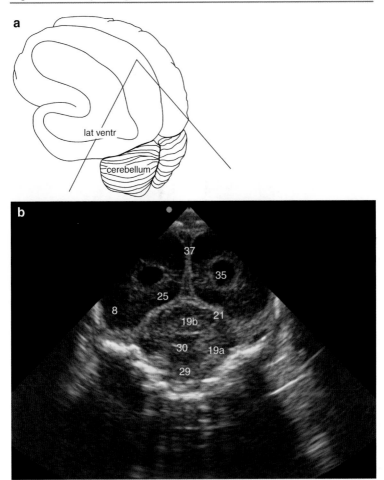

Fig. 12.3 (**a**) Coronal view, using posterior fontanel as acoustic window. (**b**) Ultrasound scan of coronal view, using posterior fontanel as acoustic window (GA 26 + 5 weeks, PMA 27 + 1 weeks)

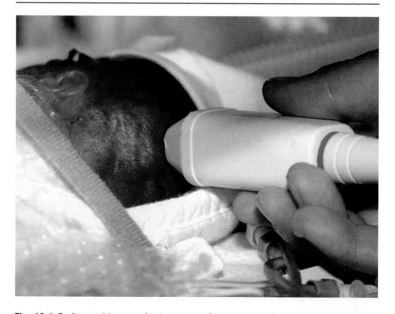

Fig. 12.4 Probe position to obtain a sagittal view, using the posterior fontanel as acoustic window. The marker (not shown here) is on the top of the probe, pointing towards the cranium

Legends of Corresponding Numbers in Ultrasound Scans

  8. Temporal lobe
 15. Choroid plexus
 16. Thalamus
 20. Temporal horn of lateral ventricle

 22. Parietal lobe
 25. Occipital lobe
 26. Calcarine fissure
 35. Occipital horn of lateral ventricle

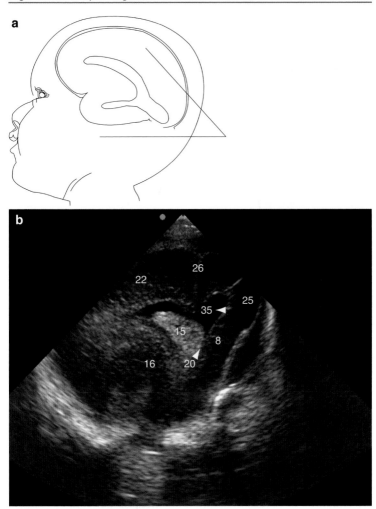

Fig. 12.5 (**a**) Parasagittal view, using posterior fontanel as acoustic window. (**b**) Ultrasound scan of parasagittal view through the right lateral ventricle, using posterior fontanel as acoustic window (GA 26 + 5 weeks, PMA 27 + 1 weeks, same infant as in Fig. 12.3b)

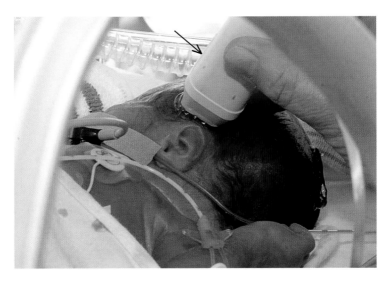

Fig. 13.1 Probe position, using the left temporal window (*arrow* indicates marker)

Legends of Corresponding Numbers in Ultrasound Scans

1. Interhemispheric fissure
8. Temporal lobe
12. → Third ventricle
18. → Mesencephalic aqueduct

19a. Cerebellar hemisphere
20. Temporal horn of lateral ventricle
27. Mesencephalon
33. Interpeduncular fossa

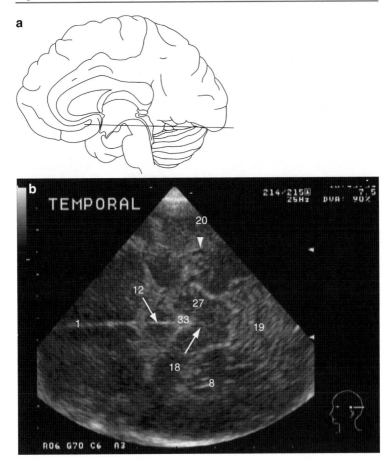

Fig. 13.2 (**a**) Transverse view, using temporal window. (**b**) Ultrasound scan of transverse view, using temporal window (GA and PMA 29 + 3 weeks). (**c**) Ultrasound scan of transverse view, using temporal window. By applying colour Doppler, the circle of Willis is shown (GA 27 weeks, PMA 29 + 4 weeks). *Arrow* indicates anterior cerebral artery, *long arrow* indicates middle cerebral artery and *arrowhead* indicates internal carotid artery

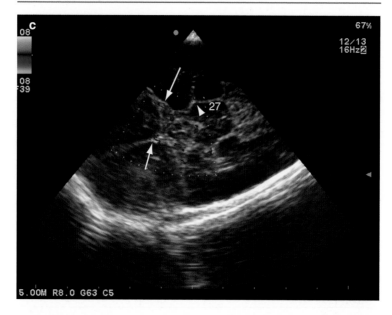

Fig. 13.2 (continued)

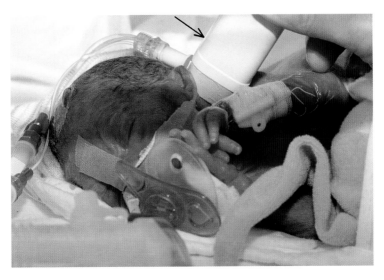

Fig. 14.1 Probe position to obtain coronal view, using the left mastoid fontanel as the acoustic window (*arrow* indicates marker)

G. Meijler, *Neonatal Cranial Ultrasonography*,
DOI 10.1007/978-3-642-21320-5_14,
© Springer-Verlag Berlin Heidelberg 2012

Legends of Corresponding Numbers in Ultrasound Scans

19a. Cerebellar hemisphere

19b. Cerebellar vermis

28. Pons

30. Fourth ventricle

31. Cisterna magna

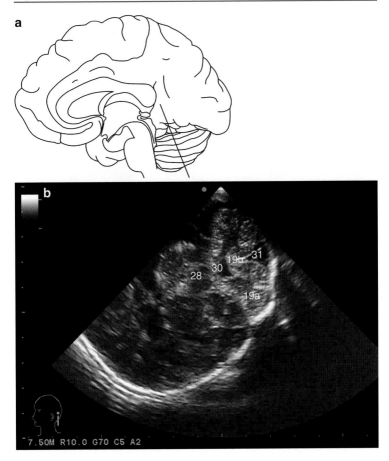

Fig. 14.2 (**a**) Coronal view, using mastoid fontanel as acoustic window. (**b**) Ultrasound scan of coronal view, using mastoid fontanel as acoustic window (GA 36 + 2 weeks, PMA 36 + 3 weeks). Note that the cerebellar hemisphere further away from the probe shows fewer details than the hemisphere closest to the probe (this is normal and should not be confused with pathological changes)

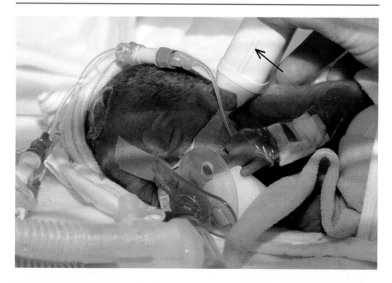

Fig. 14.3 Probe position to obtain transverse view, using the left mastoid fontanel as the acoustic window (*arrow* indicates marker)

Legends of Corresponding Numbers in Ultrasound Scans

8. Temporal lobe
19a. Cerebellar hemisphere
19b. Cerebellar vermis

25. Occipital lobe
30. → Fourth ventricle
31. Cisterna magna

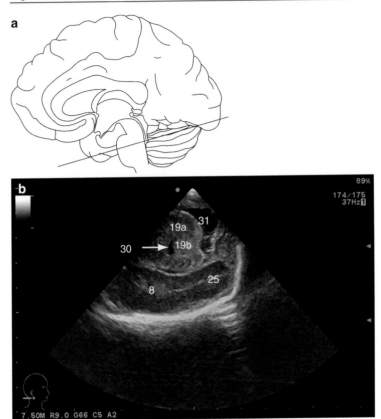

Fig. 14.4 (**a**) Transverse view, using mastoid fontanel as acoustic window. (**b**) Ultrasound scan of transverse view, using mastoid fontanel as acoustic window (GA 25 + 4 weeks, PMA 25 + 5 weeks)

Index

G. Meijler, *Neonatal Cranial Ultrasonography*,
DOI 10.1007/978-3-642-21320-5,
© Springer-Verlag Berlin Heidelberg 2012